CLINICAL AND PROCEDURAL SKILLS FOR MRCS PART B

Mr. Andrew Miller, MBBCh, BSc, MRCS
Lead Author and Editor
Convenor - Cardiff Clinical and Procedural Skills Course
Speciality Registrar - Trauma and Orthopaedic Surgery
Frenchay Hospital, Bristol

Professor Stuart Enoch, MBBS, MRCSEd, PGCert (Med Sci), MRCS (Eng), Ph.D
Editor
Programme Director, Doctors Academy Group, Cardiff, UK
Convenor - Cardiff MRCS Courses
Visiting Professor – Dept. of Biomedical Engineering, NI University, India

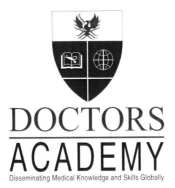

DOCTORS ACADEMY
Disseminating Medical Knowledge and Skills Globally

1st Edition, January 2014, Doctors Academy Publications, Cardiff

ALL RIGHTS RESERVED

1st Edition, January 2014, Doctors Academy Publications

Electronic versions published at	:	Doctors Academy, PO Box 4283 Cardiff, CF14 8GN, United Kingdom
Print version printed and published at	:	Abbey Bookbinding and Print Co., Unit 3, Gabalfa Workshops, Clos Menter, Cardiff CF14 3AY
ISBN	:	*978-93-80573-25-0*
Cover page Design	:	Sreekanth S.S
Type Setting	:	Lakshmi Sreekanth
Contact	:	publishing@doctorsacademy.org.uk

CLINICAL AND PROCEDURAL SKILLS FOR MRCS PART B

Andrew Miller

Stuart Enoch

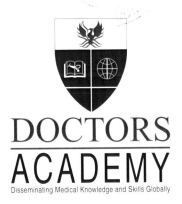

DOCTORS
ACADEMY
Disseminating Medical Knowledge and Skills Globally

1st Edition, January 2014, Doctors Ac.

i

Mr. Adam Bennett, BSc, MBBCh, MRCS
Speciality Registrar in Urology
Gloucester Royal Hospital, Gloucester

Dr. David Hepburn, MBBCh, FRCA
Speciality Registrar in Anaesthesiology
Royal Glamorgan Hospital, Llantrisant

Ms. Fran Parkinson, BSc, MBBCh, MRCS
Core Trainee in Surgery
Morriston Hospital, Swansea
Honorary Surgical Education Fellow, Doctors Academy

Ms. Karen Au-Yeung, BSc, MBBCh (Hons), MRCS (Eng)
Registrar in General Surgery
Stepping Hill Hospital, Stockport

Mr. Neil Trent, MBBCh, MRCS
Specialist Trainee in Urology
University of Wales Hospital, Cardiff

Mr. Nicholas Marsden, BSc, MBBCh, MRCS
Speciality Registrar in Plastic Surgery
Morriston Hospital, Swansea

Mr. Tom Evans, MBBCh, MRCS
Core Trainee in General and Paediatric Surgery
Prince Charles Hospital, Merthyr Tydfil
Honorary Surgical Education Fellow, Doctors Academy

PREFACE

In the Intercollegiate MRCS Examination, candidates are required to demonstrate competency in clinical and procedural skills that are relevant at the level of a junior surgical trainee. The stations are marked against a set of criteria that takes into consideration the four domains (broad content areas) - knowledge, skills, competencies and professional characteristics – which map to the General Medical Council's Good Medical Practice.

This component of the exam will test the candidate's capacity to apply sound basic science/clinical knowledge in a practical context. It will also test the candidate's ability to perform practical tasks related to surgery that requires manual dexterity, hand-eye coordination and visual/spatial awareness. In addition, this part of the exam will test aspects such as capacity, consent, theatre safety, WHO checklist and principles of safe surgery. The clinical and procedural skills may make up to about 15-20% of the overall marks in the exam.

Each chapter in this book is laid out in a format similar to a station as tested in the exam. It provides a clinical scenario/setting, important things not to miss, talk through, equipment required, one accepted way to perform the procedure and a sample mark scheme. There are some relevant questions and answers at the end of each chapter, which will help the user to prepare with a colleague in the run up to the exam.

It needs to borne in mind that this book does not intend to teach the user to simply perform the procedures, as they are mostly common tasks junior surgical trainees carry out on a day-to-day basis. Rather, it is a resource that helps the user to be informed of what is expected of them in the exam and flagging up important points that should not be missed.

In the exam, we strongly suggest that the candidate reads the scenario carefully to understand the precise nature of the task. As a general rule, in stations that involve patient/actor interaction, introducing oneself with full name and position and obtain verbal consent are important. Most tasks may be simple to perform but the exam is about demonstrating to the examiner that one is safe, meticulous, has the required knowledge and skill, and able is to interact with the patient (actor) at the same time. If one is asked to perform a procedure on a patient who is already under general anaesthetic, introduction to the patient might not be relevant but it is essential to state that the person undertaking the procedure would like to confirm the identity of the patient, checks the consent form, inspects if the surgical site has been marked and carries out the WHO checklist. All of the above can be done with a well-rehearsed statement in a very little time, securing good marks and allowing to quickly proceed to the task at hand. This concept is reinforced throughout the book.

We wish the user of this book all the very best in the exam and career.

Good luck!

Andrew Miller
Stuart Enoch

CONTENTS

ABBREVIATIONS

A&E	-	Accident and Emergency
AAA	-	Acute Abdominal Aneurysm
ABG	-	Arterial Blood Gas
ASA	-	American Society of Anesthesiologists
ATN	-	Acute Tubular Necrosis
ATLS	-	Advanced Trauma Life Support
AV	-	Arteriovenous
BAPRAS	-	British Association of Plastic, Reconstructive and Aesthetic Surgeons
BOA	-	British Orthopaedic Association
BP	-	Blood Pressure
BPM	-	Beats per Minute
BTS	-	British Thoracic Society
Ch	-	Channel
COPD	-	Chronic Obstructive Pulmonary Disease
CPR	-	Cardiopulmonary Resuscitation
CSII	-	Continuous Subcutaneous Insulin Infusion
CSF	-	Cerebrospinal Fluid
CSU	-	Catheter Specimen of Urine
CT	-	Computerised Tomography
DVT	-	Deep Venous Thrombosis
eGFR	-	estimated Glomerular Filtration Rate
ENT	-	Ear, Nose and Throat
FBC	-	Full Blood Count
FiO2	-	Fraction of Inspired Oxygen
FNA	-	Fine Needle Aspiration
GCS	-	Glasgow Coma Score
GMC	-	General Medical Council
HCA	-	Health Care Assistant
HCO_3^-	-	Bicarbonate
Hz	-	Hertz
HIV	-	Human Immunodeficiency Virus
HR	-	Heart Rate
ICP	-	Intracranial Pressure
ITU	-	Intensive Therapy Unit
IV	-	Intravenous
KCL	-	Potassium Chloride
kHz	-	Kilohertz
LA	-	Local Anaesthetic
LP	-	Lumbar Puncture
MMSE	-	Mini Mental State Examination

NCEPOD	-	National Confidential Enquiry into Patient Outcome and Death
NHS	-	National Health Service
NICE	-	National Institute for Clinical Excellence
NRCS	-	National Research Council System
ODP	-	Operation Department Personnel
pCO_2	-	Partial Pressure of Carbon Dioxide
pO_2	-	Partial Pressure of Oxygen
RR	-	Respiratory Rate
RSTL	-	Relaxed Skin Tension Lines
SHO	-	Senior House Officer
SSI	-	Surgical Site Infection
U&E	-	Urea and Electrolytes
USP	-	Universal Surgical Precautions
WHO	-	World Health Organisation

1st Edition, January 2014, Doctors Academy Publications, Cardiff

| Chapter | 1 | **Arterial Blood Gas Sampling** |

Scenario

You are the on-call Surgical SHO and have been asked by the General Surgical Consultant to perform an arterial blood gas sample on Mrs. Green who is suffering from biliary sepsis. Please perform the task and interpret the results appropriately.

Important points not to miss

As with all procedural stations you will receive marks for your communication skills, understanding of patient safety issues and for performing the task itself. It is essential that you obtain verbal consent for the procedure, perform "Allen's test" and check for any relative contraindications such as coagulopathies. Occasionally candidates are not provided with pre-loaded heparinised syringes and will have to demonstrate how to prepare a syringe themselves.

Talk through

An arterial blood gas (ABG) sample helps to assess the respiratory and metabolic function of a patient. It allows the clinician to make a fairly good clinical assessment about the patient's respiratory function by measuring the partial pressure of oxygen and carbon dioxide. In addition, the ABG results can provide evidence of metabolic dysfunction as well as compensation on the metabolic or respiratory side.

Indications

The indications are extremely broad but arterial sampling should be considered in any acutely unwell patient or any patient with respiratory compromise. Lactate, haemoglobin and some electrolytes are often also provided by some point of care blood gas analysers.

Preparation

Tell the examiner that you would wash your hands prior to approaching the patient. Introduce yourself, state your role and confirm the identity of the patient. Explain what you intend to do and the common complications of this procedure such as pain, bleeding and bruising. Obtain consent from the patient.

Ask screening questions

- Which is the dominant hand?
- Is the patient allergic to latex?

- Anticoagulant use.

The radial artery at the wrist is the easiest to feel and the most accessible. Avoid the site if it appears to be infected, inflamed or scarred. Although an arterial blood sample is commonly obtained from the radial artery, other large limb vessels such as the femoral artery are viable alternatives.

If the ABG is obtained from the wrist, perform Allen's test before sampling:
- Occlude both the radial and ulnar arteries simultaneously with both hands.
- Ask the patient to raise the hand while still occluding the vessels.
- Ask the patient to open and close the fist gently until pallor of the palm is evident.
- Release the ulnar artery.
- Reperfusion should take less than 8 seconds (Positive Allen's test).
- If there is ulnar collateral circulation you can proceed with sampling.

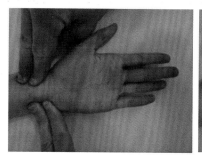

Figure 1.1: Allen's test: First occlude both radial and ulnar arteries and ask the patient to make a clenched fist and release 10 times. This will result in pallor in the palm.

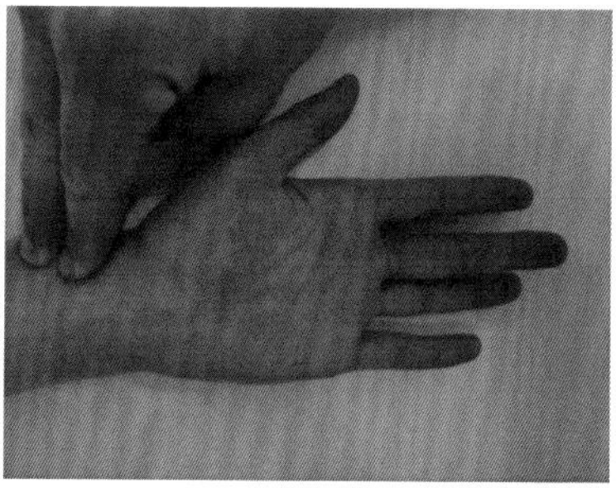

Figure 1.2: Allen's test: Release the ulnar artery only. The hand should reperfuse in <8 seconds.

Equipment
- Clean tray with sharps bin.
- Alcohol wipes or skin preparation.
- Cotton wool or gauze.
- Arterial blood gas syringe.
    Alternatively, use a 2ml syringe containing 0.1ml of 1:1,000 heparin and attach it to a 23 gauge needle (blue).
- Patient identification label.

- Blood form if the sample needs to be sent to the lab.
- Pillow or blanket on which to rest the patient's arm.
- Gloves.

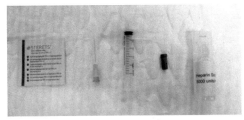

Figure 1.3: Unprepared Arterial Blood Gas Syringe

In addition, if local anaesthesia is required:

- 2ml syringe.
- 25 gauge needle (orange) for skin infiltration.
- 21 gauge needle (green) to draw up the lignocaine.
- 1% lignocaine solution.

Procedure

Support the wrist by placing the patient's arm on a pillow or blanket. Don non-sterile gloves. Extend the wrist fully after ensuring it is safe and comfortable for the patient to do so. Identify the radial artery which lies just lateral to the tendon of flexor carpi radialis. Palpate the artery just proximal to the point of maximum pulsation with your non-dominant hand. Sterilise the skin using an alcohol wipe, allow it to dry and do not re-palpate. Offer the patient local anaesthetic at this point as this procedure can be painful. With the dominant hand, hold the syringe like a pen. Insert the needle at a 45 to 60° angle with the bevel facing upwards while palpating the artery with the other hand. Advasnce the needle slowly until a flash of blood is seen in the hub of the needle. Most syringes do not require aspiration as the pressure within the artery will fill the syringe. Arterial blood is usually bright red in colour and fills the syringe quickly in a pulsatile fashion. Collect 1 to 2ml of blood, remove the needle and place it immediately in the sharps bin. Elevate the arm and ask the patient to apply firm pressure to the puncture site for 5 minutes.

Complete the procedure

Expel any air bubbles from the syringe and seal it with the cap provided. Label the syringe and roll the syringe in the palms of your hand for about 10 seconds to ensure heparin mixing. The sample should be analysed immediately or sent to the laboratory for analysis within 15 minutes of collection. If this is not possible, the sample needs to be placed in an ice bag.

Provide clinical information on the request form including:

- Full patient details-
  - Name.
  - Date of Birth.

        ‣   Hospital number.
        ‣   Address.

- FiO_2.
- Patient's temperature.

Dispose equipment into a yellow bag. Check the puncture site for complications such as haematoma. Offer to document the procedure in the notes.

Sample mark scheme

Introduction and verbal consent	0	1	2
Performs Allen's test	0	1	2
Checks for contraindication; e.g., fistula or anticoagulation	0	1	2
Gathers equipment	0	1	
Washes hands	0	1	
Dons gloves	0	1	
Identifies radial artery	0	1	
Cleans site and uses aseptic technique	0	1	2
Offers local anaesthetic	0	1	
Prepares syringe	0	1	2
Inserts needle at an appropriate site and correct angle	0	1	
Discards sharps	0	1	
Removes air from syringe	0	1	
Fills out request form correctly (patient demographics, FiO_2, temperature)	0	1	2

FOLLOW ON QUESTIONS

Please interpret the following results in relation to the clinical scenario

Normal Values

pH:	7.35 to 7.45
pO_2:	11 to 13kPa
pCO_2:	4.5 to 6kPa
BE (base excess):	-2 to +2 mmol/L
HCO^{3-}:	22 to 26 mEq/L

Q1. You are called to the ward to review a 73-year-old lady who is day one post total hip replacement. The nursing staff are concerned that she is less responsive. Her blood pressure is 127/90, Respiratory rate is 8 and Heart rate is 89 bpm. Please interpret these results and suggest a likely cause.

pH 7.15
pO_2 11.1 kPa
pCO_2 7.3 kPa
BE -1 mmol/L
HCO^{3-} 24 mEq/L

A1. The blood gas results demonstrate a reduced pH suggesting an acidaemia. There is no metabolic component to this as the base excess and bicarbonate are both normal. However, the pCO2 is raised suggesting a respiratory cause. This is therefore a respiratory acidosis without metabolic compensation. CO_2 accumulates due to hypoventilation. The most likely cause in this scenario is opiate overdose or central nervous system depression from a cerebrovascular accident.

Q2. You are asked to assess a 67-year-old smoker in pre-assessment clinic who is due for an elective hernia repair. The surgical nurse practitioner has performed an arterial blood gas as she is concerned his oxygen saturations is 91%. Please interpret these results and suggest a likely cause.

pH 7.42
pO2 9.4 kPa
pCO2 7.8 kPa
BE +9 mmol/L
HCO^{3-} 32 mEq/L

A2. The pO_2 is reduced and the pCO_2 is increased suggesting a type 2 respiratory failure. The base excess and bicarbonate are both raised but the pH is within normal limits. This is a typical picture of respiratory acidosis with metabolic compensation. In this scenario it is most likely to due to chronic hypoventilation and this patient is likely to have undiagnosed chronic obstructive pulmonary disease (COPD).

Q3. You are asked by the emergency consultant to perform a blood gas on the patient who has been involved in a road traffic accident. He is intubated and a CT scan demonstrates an open book pelvic fracture. His blood pressure is 58/40, heart rate is 140 bpm and oxygen saturation is un-recordable. Please interpret these results and suggest a likely cause.

pH 7.21
pO_2 11.5
pCO_2 5.0 kPa
BE −11 mmol/l
HCO^{3-} 14 mEq/L

A3. The pH is reduced indicating an acidaemia, pO_2 and pCO_2 are normal. Base excess and bicarbonate are markedly reduced suggesting a metabolic cause. This is metabolic acidosis without any respiratory compensation. In this scenario, the most likely cause is an acute lactic acidosis from hypovolaemia.

Q4. Your consultant has asked you to perform an arterial blood gas on a patient who is awaiting a gastrectomy. Please interpret these results and suggest a likely cause.

pH 7.51
pO_2 12 kPa
pCO_2 5.3 kPa
BE +12 mmol/l
HCO^{3-} 34 mEq/L

A4. The pH is increased suggesting an alkalosis. There is no respiratory component as the pO_2 and pCO_2 are normal. The base excess and serum bicarbonate are increased indicating a metabolic cause. This is metabolic alkalosis caused by excessive vomiting secondary to a gastric outflow obstruction.

Q5. How is metabolic acidosis subdivided? Please give examples of each

A5. Metabolic acidosis is subdivided or classified according to the anion gap.

Anion gap = $([Na^+] + [K^+]) − ([Cl^-] + [HCO^{3-}])$

Normal anion gap is <11 mEq/L and is due to a loss of bicarbonate compensated by a rise in chloride ions.
- Pancreatic fistulas.
- Gastrointestinal losses e.g., diarrhoea.
- Renal Tubular Acidosis.
- Carbonic anhydrase inhibitors.

Increased anion gap is >11 mEq/L and is due to accumulation of acid. Bicarbonate is consumed to balance the acid accumulation but there is no concurrent rise in chloride ions.
- Lactic Acidosis.
- Ketoacidosis (diabetes, alchoholism, starvation).
- Toxins e.g., salicylate, ethylene glycol, methanol.
- Accumulation of phosphoric or sulphuric acid in those with poor renal function.

Further Reading

Cowley N, Owen A, Bion J. Interpreting arterial blood gas results BMJ 2013;346:f16

Chapter 2 — Cannulation of a High Risk patient

Scenarios

1. A 25-year-old male intravenous drug user presents with a right sided groin abscess. He is seen by the on-call surgical SpR who lists him for an incision and drainage in theatre. He asks if you could kindly cannulate the patient and take bloods (FBC, U&Es, coagulation, group and save). He will also require intravenous fluids prescribing as he will be nil by mouth.

2. You are the on-call surgical core trainee at a trauma call. Please cannulate this patient, take blood and order the appropriate investigations. What fluids would you prescribe and why? What would be your plan of action from here?

Important points not to miss

As always, introduce yourself and get verbal consent. Cannulation is a simple task to perform, however this station is also about proving to the examiner that you are safe and able to interact with the patient at the same time. Be prepared for an actor playing the part of a patient and accusing you of trying to test them for HIV or drugs against their wishes.

Talk through

Indications for cannulation

- Administration of intravenous fluids - hydration.
- Administration of intravenous medications/contrast agents.
- Administration of blood products.
- Parenteral nutrition.
- Emergency access –trauma scenarios.

Equipment

- Disposable Tourniquet.
- Cannula.
  - 14Ch – Orange – 315mls/min.
  - 16Ch – Grey – 210mls/min.
  - 18Ch – Green – 110mls/min.
  - 20Ch – Pink – 65mls/min.
  - 22Ch – Blue – 25mls/min.
- Alcohol/Chlorhexidine swab.

- 10ml syringe with 0.9% Normal Saline.
- Cannula dressing.
- Personal protective equipment.
- Sharps bin and equipment tray.

Preparation
Tell the examiner that you would wash your hands prior to setting up your equipment. Choose an appropriate sized cannula as indicated by the clinical situation (*Table 2.1*).

Prepare 10mL of 0.9% normal saline flush in a 10mL syringe. Introduce yourself and include your full name and grade. Ask to check the patient's identity, *"Can I just check you are….. and what is your date of birth?"* Explain what you are about to do, why and what the complications are. The patient must give verbal or implied consent for the procedure. Position yourself and the patient, and select an appropriate vein. It can often be helpful to allow the patient's arm to hang over the side of the bed in order to distend the veins or offer to warm the patient's hands. In general, the veins on the dorsum of the hand should be used and the antecubital fossa should be reserved for trauma or emergency situations.

Procedure
Apply the tourniquet and offer to don two pairs of gloves for high risk patients. Sterilise the skin with an alcohol wipe and allow it to dry. Do not re-palpate. Check the cannula, apply skin traction and insert cannula until flashback is seen. Flatten off the angle of your approach and advance while removing the needle. Place the needle in the sharps bin. If a blood sample is required, it can be taken from the cannula at this point using a syringe or vacutainer. Release the tourniquet and occlude the vein above the level of cannulation.

Position the hub on the end of the cannula. Flush with 10ml normal saline ensuring that no resistance is felt. Apply the appropriate cannula dressing with the time and date of insertion written on it.

Dispose off all equipment into a yellow bag. Wash your hands. Offer to document date, time and site of insertion in the patient notes.

Colour	Size	Flow Rate	Situation
Blue	22G	25mls/min	Slow IV fluids and IV medications in patients with difficult veins
Pink	20G	65mls/min	Maintenance IV fluids and IV medications
Green	18G	110mls/min	Non-urgent blood transfusion / injection of contrast for imaging
Grey	16G	210mls/min	Shocked patients, massive blood loss
Orange / Brown	14G	315mls/min	Shocked patients requiring urgent resuscitation, massive blood loss requiring urgent blood volume replacement

Table 2.1: Types of cannulae and indications for cannulation

Usual sites for peripheral access
- Basilic vein.
- Cephalic vein.
- Median cubital vein.

High risk patients
- Universal precautions.
  ‣ Double glove.
  ‣ Eye wear.
  ‣ Gowns.
Masks if required
- Safe sharps practice.
  ‣ Sharps bin close by.
  ‣ Never re-sheath used needle.

Complications
- Phebitis – Infection; chemical irritant solutions.
- Extravasation in malpositioned cannula.
- Occlusion.
- Haematoma formation after cannula removal.

Sample mark scheme

Introduction and orientation – Checks identity, explains procedure, gains consent and obtains information such as high risk behaviour, allergies	0	1	2
Gathers correct equipment and sharps bin. Applies protective equipment	0	1	2
Selects appropriate vein and can demonstrate anatomy	0	1	2
Applies tourniquet	0	1	
Cleans site	0	1	
Warns the patient prior to needle entry	0	1	
Inserts cannula appropriately, withdrawing needle on entry into vein	0	1	
Takes blood appropriately	0	1	2
Releases tourniquet	0	1	
Disposes off sharps correctly	0	1	
Applies dressing to cannula site	0	1	
Labels dressing with date of insertion	0	1	
Labels blood specimens appropriately – label high risk, hand written 'Group and Save' bottle after checking patient identification	0	1	2
Places in 'High Risk' bag	0	1	
Prescribes intravenous fluid correctly	0	1	

FOLLOW ON QUESTIONS

Q1. What would you do if you sustain a sharps injury?

A1.

- Encourage bleeding.
- Wash with water and soap.
- Contact occupational health department and seek their advice.
- If occupational health team is not available, then contact A&E since they have a needle stick policy.
- Contact patient involved and counsel for testing of Hepatitis B & C and HIV. Obtain blood samples from both you and the patient.
- Discuss post-exposure prophylaxis with occupational health or Consultant Microbiologist.

Q2. How would you minimise the risk of disease transmission when operating on high risk patients?

A2.

- Clear communication.
- Disposable gowns and drapes.
- Personal protective equipment.
  - Double glove.
  - Eye protection.
  - Face masks.
- Safe handling of sharps – blunt suture needles, bowls for blades etc.
- Minimise amount of staff in theatre or by the bedside.

Q3. What pre-operative fluids would you prescribe for this patient and what are the constituents of this fluid?

A3.

- Some possible options:
- 1L Normal Saline 0.9%.
  - pH 5.0.
  - 9g NaCl per litre.
  - Osmolality of 308 mOsmol/L.
  - Constituents-
    - 154 mmol/L Sodium.
    - 154 mmol/L Chloride.
- 1L Hartmanns solution.
  - pH 6.5.
  - Osmolality 279mOsmol/L.
  - Constituents-

- ‣ 131 mmol/L Sodium.
- ‣ 111 mmol/L Chloride.
- ‣ 29 mmol/L Lactate.
- ‣ 5 mmol/L Potassium.
- ‣ 2mmol/L Calcium.
- 1L 5% Dextrose.
  - ▪ Osmolality 253 mOsmol/L.
  - ▪ Constituents-
    - ‣ 278mmol/L Glucose.
    - ‣ 50g Glucose.

Q4. What is the difference between a crystalloid and colloid?

A4. A colloid is a fluid containing large insoluble molecules such as gelatin that exert an oncotic pressure and draws water into the intravascular compartment. A crystalloid is a solution containing electrolytes such as sodium, chloride and potassium in ionic form. Colloids remain in the intravascular compartment for longer as the large molecules are not immediately broken down and continue to exert an oncotic pressure. Electrolytes in crystalloid solutions can freely diffuse across a cell membrane.

Q5. What would you do if a medication extravasates into the skin?

A5.
- Stop the infusion or injection immediately, place a syringe on the end of the cannula and slowly aspirate the medication back.
- Remove the cannula and elevate the arm (leave in situ for chemotherapy agents).
- If blisters form on the arm they can be aspirated with a small gauge needle.
- If the medication is a chemotherapy agent, there are substrate specific measures that can be performed e.g., topical cooling, hyaluronidase or dexrazone injections.
- If in doubt contact plastic surgical team for advice.

Further Reading

Dougherty L (2008) Peripheral cannulation. Nursing Standard. 22, 52, 49-56.

Chapter 3 — Consent

Scenario

This patient has already been consented for a Hartmann's procedure by the consultant. You have 10 minutes to read a set of patient's notes before being asked to talk to the patient about his upcoming operation. The notes contain all the answers to the questions that the patient will ask e.g., there is a 40% chance we will not be able to reverse the stoma and there is a 10% chance of death. The patient is very distressed and is in a lot of pain.

Important points not to miss

Always introduce yourself with your full name and position. It is important to be sympathetic, talk to the patient at their eye level and act as if you are in a hospital. Offer the patient some pain relief if they are clearly distressed and ask if there is anyone else they would like to join them for the discussion.

Talk Through

Always check what the patient knows before you start talking and let them lead the conversation. If you don't know the answer or they have asked you something that is not in the notes don't be tempted to make it up or bluff your way through it. It is much more professional to say you don't know and offer to find out when you leave and come back to them with the answer.

At the end of the station ask if the patient has any further questions and suggest that they write down anything they wish to ask in the future so they don't forget. Provide the patient with your full name and grade again and make sure they know that you are happy to come back later to answer further questions.

Sample mark scheme

Introduction – Full name and position	0	1	2
Moves to patient eye level	0	1	
Asks if patient would like anyone else to join them e.g., family member	0	1	
Checks prior knowledge	0	1	2
Explains indication for procedure	0	1	2
Explains procedure in lay terms	0	1	2
Answers specific question from patients notes e.g., chance of reversal	0	1	2
Answers specific question from patients notes e.g., chance of death	0	1	2
Ensures patient understands that it is their decision and does not feel coerced	0	1	2
Suggests patient writes down further questions	0	1	2
Offers to come and discuss again at a later date	0	1	2

FOLLOW ON QUESTIONS

Q1. When do you need written consent for a procedure?

A1. Any treatment that involves "significant" risk not just operations. It is good practice to obtain written consent for even minor procedures that do not involve general anaesthetics like manipulations in the emergency department and chest drains.

The GMC states that written consent should be obtained if:

- The investigation or treatment involves significant risks
- Significant consequences for the patient's employment, social or personal life
- The treatment is part of a research programme

Q2. Must you be able to do the procedure to consent it?

A2. No. Providing you are:

- Suitably trained and qualified (i.e. a doctor or nurse)
- Have sufficient knowledge of the proposed investigation or treatment
- Understand the risks involved
- Acting in accordance with GMC Guidelines 2008

However it is the person who performs the procedure who is ultimately responsible for ensuring the patient has been counselled and consented appropriately.

Q3. Is it necessary for you provide a patient with details about all the common complications of a procedure or investigation in order to get informed consent?

A3. Yes, it is important to explain and document all the common complications and side effects of a proposed treatment, but you must also inform patients of rare complications if they would result in a "serious adverse outcome".

Q4. How can a patient inform you that they have given their consent?

A4. Consent can be written, verbal or implied. Implied consent is when a patient uses body language or actions to confirm they are happy to proceed e.g. a patient will roll up their sleeve to have a blood test

Q5. What must a patient have in order to give informed consent?

A5. The patient must have:

- Been provided with sufficient information at the time of consent.
- Understand the implications and future consequences of their decision.
- Adequate reasoning faculties i.e., Capacity.
- Come to that decision without duress or coercion.

Further Reading

Consent: Patients and doctors making decisions together. GMC Publication 2008

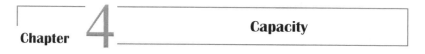

Chapter 4 | Capacity

Scenario
Please assess this lady's capacity. She is about to undergo a total hip replacement and has been consented in the pre-operative assessment clinic by your house officer.

Important points not to miss
Capacity is not the same as cognitive function but this station may be used as a surrogate marker. In this station, you will be marked for demonstrating probity, patient safety and a basic understanding of what is required to give informed consent.

Talk through
This can be a very difficult station. You may find this station disjointed and confusing. Be prepared to perform a mini mental state examination (MMSE) in this station if asked.

It is essential as with all stations that you introduce yourself to the patient in full. The actor may make it quite clear that they do not have capacity but it is up to you to demonstrate this to the examiner. It is often best to start by asking what operation they are having or if they have any questions about the operation. You can then ask what the operation entails and if they remember some of the complications or risks.

It is important to demonstrate to the examiner that you understand the components of consent. For a patient to give consent they must:
- understand the facts involved in that decision.
- appreciate the severity of the decision.
- have the ability to weigh risks and benefits.
- be able to communicate their choice.

Although cognition is not a component of capacity, by performing the MMSE you can demonstrate that the patient is unlikely to understand the facts and therefore unlikely to have capacity.

The MMSE is a set of questions with a maximum score of 30 that assesses overall cognition. A score of 25 or more suggests normal cognition, 21 to 24 is mild impairment, 10 to 20 is moderate impairment and less than or equal to 9 is severe impairment.

- Orientation to time (5)-
  - Year
  - Season
  - Date
  - Month
  - Day
- Orientation to Place (5)-
  - Country
  - County
  - City
  - Hospital
  - Floor
- Registration (3)-
  - Immediately repeat 3 unrelated items
- Attention and calculation (5)-
  - Add 7s or spell word backwards
- Recall (3)-
  - Delayed Recall of 3 items
- Language (2)-
  - Names 2 items from sight e.g. watch and pen
- Repetition (1)-
  - Repeat a sentence
- Complex command (6)-
  - Reproduce interlocking pentagons

Once you have demonstrated to the examiner that the patient does not have capacity, it is important to explain that it is inappropriate to preceed as it is an elective procedure and there is doubt over the patient's ability to give informed consent.

It looks professional if you offer to discuss your decision with the nursing staff and senior doctors before informing the patient and their family of your decision.

Sample mark scheme

Introduction – Full name and position	0	1	2
Assesses understanding of procedure	0	1	2
Performs Mini Mental State Examination			
Orientation to time	0	1	2
Orientation to place	0	1	2
Registration	0	1	2
Attention and calculation	0	1	2
Recall	0	1	2
Language	0	1	2
Repetition	0	1	2
Complex command	0	1	2

FOLLOW ON QUESTIONS

Q1. If a patient with capacity refuses treatment, you can treat them under "common law"?

A1. No, that is assault. If they were competent at the time of their decision you must accept it whether you agree or not.

Q2. In an emergency situation where a patient lacks capacity or is unable to express their wishes, can you provide any medical treatment you feel

A2. No, you can provide only what is deemed immediately necessary to save their life or to prevent a serious deterioration of their condition.

Q3. At what age is a child assumed to have capacity?

A3. Children are assumed to have capacity at 16 years of age.

Q4. What is "Gillick" Competence?

A4. "Gillick" competence is a precedent set by the case of Victoria Gillick v West Norfolk and Wisbech Area Health Authority in 1985. It states that a child under the age of 16 years old can consent to a procedure providing they have adequate maturity and understanding.

Q5. Who should you seek consent from if a child (<16) doesn't have capacity i.e. is not Gillick competent?

A5. Someone who has "Parental Responsibility". This is most often the child's biological mother or father but it may also be a step parent, foster parent or even teacher in some situations.

Q6. Can you override a competent child's refusal of a procedure?

A6. Yes, a parent can override a competent child's decision not to have a treatment that is in their best interest. This is however a complex legal area and should be discussed with a lawyer and is not the case in Scotland.
A doctor can also override a parents wish not to have their child treated by applying for "Parens Patriae" through the courts.

Q7. What are the specific considerations when treating a Jehovah's witness?

A7. Most Jehovah's witnesses refuse blood products of any kind including pre donation. However, many would consider organ transfer acceptable. It is essential that a discussion is had with each patient to ensure that we fully understand their individual beliefs.

Q8. In an emergency situation can you give a Jehovah's Witness any blood products?

A8. If an adult patient has capacity and has refused blood products then their decision must be accepted. If the patient is not able to give informed consent and there is no advanced directive or living will available then the doctor should treat the patient in their best interests. This is irrespective of the opinion of the patient's friends or family.

Q9. Can you give a child blood products against their wishes or their parents' wishes?

A9. If haemorrhage cannot be controlled and a child needs blood to save their life then it should be given. A surgeon who allows a minor to die where death could have been avoidable can be subject to prosecution. However, if time allows, advice should always be sought from medical indemnity providers, senior colleagues and the trust legal department before proceeding.

Further Reading

- *0-18 years: Guidance for the doctors. GMC Publication 2007*
- *Code of Practice for The Surgical Management of Jehovah's Witnesses. Royal College of Surgeons of England 2002*

Chapter 5 — Debridement of a Contaminated Wound

Scenario

You are the on-call orthopaedic trainee. A 36-year-old patient has been referred to yourself with a 10 x 6cm traumatic wound to his left thigh after a mountain biking accident. He is normally fit and well with no other injuries. The wound is contaminated and requires surgical debridement in theatre. The patient is undergoing general anaesthetic but unfortunately your SpR has just been called away to deal with an emergency and has asked you to debride this wound.

Important things not to miss

As with all stations in the exam, read the scenario carefully to understand exactly what your task is. As stated in the task, the patient is under a general anaesthetic and hence introduction to the patient is not relevant. However, don't forget to state you would like to confirm the identity of the patient, best done by asking to see the wristband. Now ask to see the consent form and check that the surgical site has been marked. You should ask to see any X-rays of the limb to check for obvious fractures or foreign bodies. At this point you should then state that you would carry out the WHO checklist with all staff in theatre. All of the above can be done with a well-rehearsed statement in very little time, securing you good marks and allowing you to quickly proceed to the task at hand.

Talk through

This is a common skill station in the Intercollegiate Basic Surgical Skills course and so should be considered as a station where marks can be easy to obtain if you have a set routine. You will likely be presented with a cut of meat (e.g. a turkey or lamb leg) in which a simulated traumatic and contaminated wound has been produced. The fact that the scenario tells you the patient is under general anaesthetic means that you won't be expected to communicate with the patient, however there will be plenty of marks to gain prior to actually debriding the wound. Candidates will be expected to gather the appropriate equipment, undertake the procedure and then answer any follow on questions. The mistake is to panic that you won't have time to finish the debridement and jump straight into it. As with all of the clinical skills stations, there will be easy marks to be gained from a few well-rehearsed statements before starting.

Equipment

Due to time restraints, the correct equipment will be provided for you and the patient (chicken/lamb) is already prepared and draped. However, be prepared to clean and drape the wound if asked. Equipment that you may require includes:

- Sterile gloves and gown.
- Skin preparation solution (Iodine or Chlorhexidine in alcohol).
- Sterile drapes.
- Irrigation fluid (saline).
- 50ml Syringe.
- Scalpel and no.10 or 15 blade.
- Scissors – curved iris or straight tips.
- Toothed forceps.
- Non-toothed forceps.
- Dressing gauze (other suitable packing).

Procedure
In this scenario with a traumatic wound to the limb, you should state that you would like to perform the debridement under tourniquet control, to reduce bleeding and allow thorough examination of important structures (neurovascular, tendons etc). You will not be expected to apply a tourniquet in the scenario but be sure to mention it.

You will be supplied with a simulated contaminated wound, which will likely have gross contaminants and foreign material in the wound. After initial inspection, any obvious gross contaminants or foreign bodies should be removed with non-toothed forceps. Gentle wound irrigation using normal saline and a 50ml syringe, and a damp gauze can then be used to wipe away any finer contaminants.

Following this, a thorough and detailed wound inspection should be carried out. It is best to have a method for inspection that you can easily describe, such as clockwise from superficial to deep, so that no part of the wound is left unexamined. You should be seen to palpate and probe the wound to check for hidden cavities and degloving injuries.

Adequate debridement requires excision of all necrotic or non-viable tissue including skin, subcutaneous fat, muscle and even bone. Again, in the same way that you explored the wound, systematically debride all unhealthy tissue using a combination of blunt and sharp dissection (using a scalpel and scissors), aiming to preserve important structures already identified. Ensure all non-viable tissue is excised – too little debridement is worse than too much.

Finally, thoroughly washout the wound again with saline and a 50ml syringe, until the wound is clean of contaminants and necrotic tissue. State that you would leave the wound open and either pack the wound with Betadine soaked gauze, or if available, use a negative pressure dressing. When you have finished with your equipment, be sure to dispose all sharps appropriately into a sharps bin.

Post-operative instructions & follow up
Once you are happy you have completed the debridement and the wound is dressed appropriately, you should state that you would now like to write a detailed operation note, including your post-operative plan.

Ensure you mention the need for antibiotics, initially a broad-spectrum empirical antibiotic (e.g., Co-amoxiclav) as per hospital guidelines. Also, mention the need to check the patient's tetanus status, as in the case with all traumatic wounds.

Finally, ensure you make plans for a second look at the wound in 24-48 hours, either on the ward or in theatre.

Sample mark scheme

Checks patient identity	0	1	
Checks mark & consent	0	1	2
Checks for X-Ray	0	1	
Performs WHO checklist	0	1	
Chooses appropriate equipment	0	1	
Prepares / drapes / scrubs	0	1	
Applies tourniquet	0	1	
Removes gross contaminants	0	1	
Thoroughly examines and inspects the extent of the wound	0	1	2
Identifies important structures (NV structures, tendons)	0	1	2
Adequately debrides all necrotic tissue	0	1	2
Irrigates wound appropriately	0	1	
Dresses wound appropriately (wound pack / negative pressure)	0	1	
Disposes sharps appropriately	0	1	
Indicates need for antibiotics	0	1	
Indicates need to check tetanus status	0	1	

FOLLOW ON QUESTIONS

Q1. What is the importance of debriding a necrotic wound?

A1.
- Necrotic tissue may serve as a source of nutrients for bacteria, particularly anaerobes such as Bacteroides species and *Clostridium perfringens*.
- Devitalised tissue acts as a physical barrier to healing.
- Devitalised tissue can prevent the effectiveness of topical preparations such as antimicrobial agents.
- The presence of devitalised tissue within the wound may mask or mimic signs of infection.
- The presence of necrotic tissue within the wound may prevent the surgeon from gaining an accurate picture of the extent of tissue damage, thus inhibiting the ability to assess the wound correctly.

Q2. What do you know about Necrotising fasciitis?

A2. Necrotising fasciitis is a surgical emergency, characterized by a rapidly progressive, necrotising infection along the fascial layers and subcutaneous tissue. The infection spreads rapidly from the subcutaneous tissue along the superficial and deep fascial planes, leading to extensive underlying tissue necrosis whilst the skin may appear relatively normal in the early stages of the disease. Later, once the skin becomes deprived of its blood and nerve supply, it also undergoes necrosis. It is a life-threatening condition where the patient may present in a state of septic shock.

It is commonly caused by a synergistic, polymicrobiol infection (anaerobes and aerobes). Monomicrobial infection is usually caused by haemolytic group A streptococcus.

Management includes:
- Aggressive resuscitation and invasive monitoring.
- Early antibiotic therapy, initial broad spectrum empirical therapy, adjusted under the direction of a microbiologist and results of cultures.
- Emergency and aggressive surgical debridement of all involved tissue.
- Wound packing.
- Early and regular re-exploration +/- further debridement.

Q3. How would you distinguish between necrotic and viable tissue?

A3.

Tissue	Necrotic	Viable
Fat	Dull Grey/brown/dark	Shiny/glistening yellow
Fascia	Dull Grey/dark	Shiny/glistening white
Muscle	Brown/dark red Does not contract	Red/pink Contracts
All tissue	Insensate Does not bleed malodourous	Sensate Bleeding tissue No/little odour

Table 5.1: Differences between necrotic and viable tissue

Further Reading

- *Intercollegiate Basic Surgical Skills Course Manual. Royal College of Surgeons of England. Fourth Edition 2007.*

- *Guidelines for wound debridement (open lower limb fractures) BAPRAS and BOA Publication 2009.*

| Chapter | 6 | **Electrosurgery (diathermy) and Tourniquets** |

Scenario

Questions about diathermy and tourniquets are often part of the critical care stations but can also be asked as follow on questions after the "suturing skills" and "removal of a naevus" stations.

Important things not to miss

It is essential that you know the definition, basic principles and understand the patient safety issues surrounding their use.

Talk through

You may be provided with a selection of leads, pads and tourniquets. You must be able to identify equipment that is commonly used in theatre. This can be daunting if you have not seen them before. Next time you are in theatre take a few minutes to familiarise yourself with the basics of diathermy and tourniquets.

Electrosurgery (diathermy)

Electrosurgery or diathermy is used in almost every surgical speciality and you must have a basic understanding of the key concepts. Diathermy comes from the Greek phrase "to heat through".

It uses high frequency alternating current to produce heat in order to cut or coagulate tissue. Current can either travel in a single direction (direct) or change direction (alternating). The number of times an alternating current changes direction or polarity in a second is referred to as the frequency and is measured in Hertz (Hz). Human muscle will depolarise and contract if a current of less than 10,000 Hertz (10kHz) passes through it. Diathermy, therefore, uses a current more than 500, 000 Hz (500 kHz) to allow local heating of tissue without depolarising muscle.

The amount of heat produced by the electrode is directly proportional to the power produced by the generator. The ability to heat tissue is also related to the surface area of the electrode that is in contact with the patient. The tip of the cutting electrode touches only a small area of the patient and therefore the amount of current that passes into the patient per unit area is very high. This is known as a high current density and will produce high temperatures to cut tissue. In contrast, the diathermy pad has a very large area for the same amount of current. This is known as a low current density and will not cause a significant amount of heating. Problems with the initial design of diathermy pads meant that if the pad became loose the patient would be at risk of burns. Newer designs have two adhesive pads and machines will alarm if the pad is not attached correctly. In order to reduce the risk of burns it is essential that the diathermy pad is placed on well vascularised muscle, away from metal prosthesis and bone prominences.

All electrosurgery equipment is insulated to prevent leaking of electrical current to the surrounding tissue or surgeon. It is, however, impossible to prevent 100% of this leakage. As the frequency increases, the amount of radiation through the insulator also increases and leads to problems called 'capacitance'. Electrical current will pass through the path of least resistance and if the diathermy is activated while not in contact with the patient the energy may pass through the insulation to the surgeon's glove. This same concept applies to why diathermy leads must not be wrapped around towel clips and why the insulation of the handpiece must not be in contact with the patient's tissues while the diathermy is active.

It is also important to understand the difference between generator output modes. Most generators will have the ability to cut, coagulate and often have a blend function. In order to cut tissue, a constant alternating current is used with produces rapid heating and tissue vaporisation. Coagulation is achieved by interrupting (or modulating) the current which produces slower heating and shrinking of the tissues. Blend is a combination of 'cut and coagulate' modes.

Diathermy can be either monopolar or bipolar. In monopolar diathermy, current passes from a handpiece through the patient to an electrode pad. Its use is contraindicated in close proximity to a pacemaker and should not be used near vascular pedicles such as the digits or penis. In bipolar systems, the current passes between two points of the same instrument. The patient's body is excluded from the electrical circuit and is therefore safe for pacemakers and vascular pedicles.

Tourniquets
Surgical tourniquets comprise of a cuff and valve system that is attached to a pump and pressure monitor. However, a tourniquet can be any material that is used to control the vasculature of a limb. They are commonly used in surgical practice to facilitate a bloodless field but also have an increasing role in trauma care, administration of regional anaesthetics and local chemotherapy.

Factors such as age, general health of the patient and pre-existing diseases such as diabetes or thickening of the arterial wall should be taken into consideration before application of the tourniquet. In fit and healthy adults, effective tourniquet pressure for upper limbs may be achieved at pressure settings of about 75-100 mmHg above the pre-operative systolic blood pressure, and double the preoperative systolic blood pressure for lower limbs. Generally, in adults, a tourniquet pressure of 180-200 mmHg is used in the upper limb (arm and 240-300 mmHg in the lower limb (thigh). In healthy adults, the maximum tourniquet time at a stretch should be 120 minutes, followed by a minimum of 10 minutes break to help reperfuse the limb (remove metabolic waste products and nourish the tissue with oxygenated blood). If further breaks are needed for reperfusion, they need to be slightly longer (15-20 minutes).

Complications of tourniquet use can be local or systemic. Local complications are caused by direct pressure on nerves, blood vessels or the skin. There is also a recognised physiological change following inflation or deflation of a tourniquet due to the relative decrease or sudden increase in available circulating volume and the metabolites released from the sequestered tissues.

Sample mark scheme

Identifies diathermy equipment and generator	0	1	2
What is the definition of electrosurgery?	0	1	2
What are the different generator outputs?	0	1	2
What is the difference between monopolar and bipolar diathermy?	0	1	2
Provide 2 complications of electrosurgery	0	1	2
Provide 2 contraindications of monopolar diathermy	0	1	2
What is the definition of a tourniquet?	0	1	2
Provide 2 uses of tourniquets	0	1	2
Provide 2 local complications	0	1	2
Provide 2 systemic complications	0	1	2

FOLLOW ON QUESTIONS

Q1. What is Diathermy?

A1. Diathermy is a surgical technique that uses a high frequency alternating current to produce a local heating effect in order to cut or coagulate tissue.

Q2. In electricity terms, what is the equation for power?

A2. Power (Watts) = Voltage (Volts) x Currents (Amps).

Q3. What is the relationship between power and heat production?

A3. The heat produced is directly proportional the power generated.

Q4. What do you understand by the term alternating current and what is the unit of frequency?

A4. An alternating current is an electrical current that changes direction (polarity) and the unit is Hertz (Number of alternations per second).

Q5. At what frequency can electrical current pass through human tissue without causing muscular stimulation?

A5. >10,000 Hertz or 10 kilohertz can pass through the body without causing neuromuscular stimulation (depolarization).

Q6. What is capacitance? Please give an example of a surgical burn from this process

A6. Capacitance is the ability of a substance to store an electrical charge. In medical terms it refers to the situation when two conductors are separated by an insulator. With high frequency currents, insulation is not 100% effective and will leak (radiate) through the insulator to the adjacent conductor.

This often occurs during non-contact activation of monopolar diathermy as the path of least resistance is through the insulation, not the air. Skin burns can occur if the insulation of the diathermy hand piece rests against the skin while cutting deep tissues. Inadvertent burns can also occur if diathermy leads are wrapped around metal clips to prevent them falling from the operating table.

Q7. What generator output modes do you know?

A7.
- Cut – An uninterrupted alternating current allows rapid heating causing vaporisation of cells.

- Coagulate – Modulated (with pauses) waveform allows dissipation of heat, evaporates water more slowly.
- Blend – a combination of the two.

Q8. What types of diathermy do you know?

A8.
- Monopolar – from the tip of the hand piece to a large pad on the patient.
- Bipolar – between the two tips of the hand piece.
- Feedback controlled e.g., ligasure - generator senses resistance and switches off the electrical current once tissues are cut.

Q9. Can you name some dangers associated with electrosurgery?

A9.
- Burns - Alternative pathways of conductance e.g., through a metal table or myocardial burns if monopolar is used in a patient with a pacemaker.
- Fire - Pools of alcohol-based skin preparation solution can ignite.
- Smoke - Carcinogenic smoke.
- Pedicles - Bipolar must not be used on pedicles such as fingers and penis.

Q10. What is a tourniquet?

A10. A tourniquet is a constricting device used to control venous and or arterial circulation to a limb.

Q11. What are the uses of a tourniquet?

A11.
- Surgical.
  - Reduce blood loss.
  - Improve surgical field.
- Anaesthetic.
  - Regional blocks e.g., Biers block.
- Medical.
  - Local administration of drugs e.g. chemotherapy for melanoma.

Q12. How long can a tourniquet be left on an extremity?

A12. In healthy adults, 2 hours is the maximum recommended time before the tourniquet is deflated for a minimum of 10 minutes to allow reperfusion of the limb.

Q13. What pressure is normally used?

A13.
- Adults
  - Upper Limb: 180 - 200 mmHg.

- Lower Limb: 240 - 300 mm Hg.
- Children
- Upper Limb: 175 +/- 30 mmHg.
- Lower Limb: 210 +/- 10 mm Hg.

Q14. What are the local complications of using a tourniquet?

A14.
- Skin lesions
  - Abrasions.
  - Bullous lesions.
- Neurapraxias
  - Radial 1:10,000 risk.
  - Sciatic 1:25,000 risk.
- Muscle Ischaemia
- Compartment syndrome following reperfusion injury
- Vascular Injuries
  - Ruptured vessels.
  - Embolisation of plaques.
- Post-tourniquet syndrome
  - Stiffness.
  - Colour change to the limb.
  - Mild weakness.
  - Paraesthesia.

Q15. What are the systemic complications of tourniquet use?

A15.
- Cardiovascular effects
  - Inflation - circulating blood volume increase as does systemic vascular resistance.
  - Deflation - sudden decrease in central venous pressure can reduce blood pressure.
  - Both of which can cause acute cardiac failure.
- Respiratory effects
  - Deflation - Transient hypercapnia (about 1kPa).
- Cerebral circulation
  - Deflation – Hypercapnia increases Intracranial pressure (ICP) and can result in a secondary brain injury.
- Metabolic changes
  - Deflation - Potassium increases (about 0.5 mmol/l).

Further Reading

Medicines and Healthcare produce regulatory Agency Guidelines Perioperative management pacemakers/ICDs. March 2006

Chapter 7 — **Fine Needle Aspiration**

Scenario
You are in the ENT clinic and have found a mass in this patient's thyroid. Your consultant has asked you to perform a Fine Needle Aspiration Biopsy and prepare some slides for histology.

Important points not to miss
Always introduce yourself, offer local anaesthetic and check the mass is not pulsatile. Although you would have never prepared a slide for histology, please ensure that you understand the essential concepts. Label the slides before the procedure as writing on wet slides can be difficult. Don't forget to take the needle off at the end of the procedure, fill the same syringe with air and then expel the contents onto the slide. Not all the slides need to be fixed.

Talk through
Fine needle aspiration is a simple, safe procedure to obtain cellular material for cytological examination and diagnosis using a 21-gauge or smaller needle. It is a simple procedure that is frequently tested in the exam as it is a commonly performed in surgical outpatient departments. Take some time to see or familiarise with this procedure before the exam.

Indications
There are no absolute indications for fine needle aspiration, but it is used commonly in the assessment of:
- Neck lumps.
- Thyroid nodules.
- Breast lumps.
- Cutaneous lumps.
- Lymph nodes.

Awareness that a core or excision biopsy is an alternate method is very important. These techniques will obtain more tissue for diagnostic purposes and provide details about the architecture of the tissue. However, they are associated with higher complication rates than fine needle aspiration.

Consent
Although written consent is not essential for fine needle aspiration, it should be considered in situations when a patient is anticoagulated or the procedure is radiologically guided.

The risk of serious complication is significantly less than 1% (around 0.05%)
- Haemorrhage.
- Haematoma.
- Seeding of tumour.
- Location specific e.g. pneumothorax in a slim patient having skin or breast sampling.

Equipment
- Small dressing pack (includes drape/gauze/gallipot).
- Sterile gloves.
- Cleaning solution (2% chlorhexidene spray).
- 21-27G needle.
- 5-20ml syringe.
- 2-3 microscope slides.
- Pencil/wax crayon.
- Fixing solution (usually ethanol based).
- Universal container (if cystic fluid present).

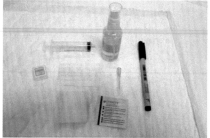

Figure 7.1: Fine Needle Aspiration Equipment

*local anaesthetic should be offered, but is likely to be more painful than the procedure.

Note: Fine needle aspiration is not commonly performed as a 'sterile' procedure, but for the purpose of this exam, treat it as such.

Positioning
This is dependant upon the area for sampling, but ensure both the patient and yourself are comfortable and you have adequate access to the area for sampling. Make sure the patient is exposed appropriately, with curtains, sheets and offer a chaperone if you deem it to be appropriate.

In both neck and breast lumps, these are both best sampled with the patient supine at 30-45°.

Procedure
Introduce yourself, confirm the patient's identity and confirm the site to be sampled. Ensure the patient understands the procedure and obtain verbal consent. Ask if the patient has any allergies, specifically latex or chlorhexidine. Position the patient and ensure dignity. Wash your hands and prepare the equipment including writing the patient's details on the slides provided (this is much easier pre-procedure).

Expose the patient adequately, protect clothing/face and use disinfectant spray. Remember, these are usually alcohol based and work by evaporation, so allow to dry. Cleanse hands with an alcohol-based agent. Don sterile gloves and drape the patient.

Ensure you examine the lump if you have not already done so. Make sure it is not pulsatile. Inform the patient they will feel a sharp sensation, but it will only take a few seconds to perform.

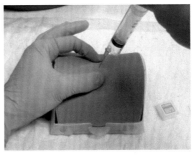

Figure 7.2: *Fine Needle Aspiration: Aspirate while passing the needle through the lesion*

Attach the needle to the syringe and advance into the lesion and aspirate. If you aspirate fluid, do so until no further fluid can be aspirated. If not, take several passes through the lesion with the syringe aspirating as you pass. Remove the needle and apply pressure to the area with gauze/cotton wool ball. Apply a dressing (a simple plaster will suffice) to the wound and allow the patient to dress.

With the needle removed, detach it from the syringe, fill the syringe with air and re-attach the needle. Empty the contents of the syringe onto a slide and quickly prepare the slides. This involves placing two slides together. This takes some practice to do effectively. Apply fixation solution to the slides and allow it

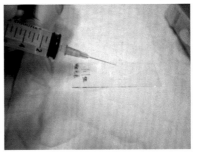

Figure 7.3: *Preparing the slides: Remove the needle, fill the syringe with air and empty the contents onto a single slide.*

to dry. One slide is usually prepared without a fixing solution

Ensure the appropriate labels are on the sample (confirm with patient). Inform them of what to do if a complication arises.

Dispose off the sharps and any other equipment in the appropriate bin.

Document the procedure

- Date and time.
- Indication.
- Consent obtained.
- Complications/Difficulties encountered, if any.

Sample mark scheme

Introduction, confirmation of patient identity	0	1	2
Professionalism	0	1	2
Explains and obtains verbal consent	0	1	2
Examines the mass	0	1	
Checks for pulsation/local structures	0	1	
Wash hands and prepares skin	0	1	
Offers local anaesthetic	0	1	
Selects appropriate equipment	0	1	2
Carries out the procedure appropriately	0	1	2
Prepares slide in the correct manner (Multiple Slides/ labelled/fixed)	0	1	2
Explains to patient post procedure			
Warns patient about risk of infection and haematoma	0	1	2
Answers relevant questions. Is it Cancer….?	0	1	2

FOLLOW ON QUESTIONS

Q1. What are the possible cytological results of the FNA?

A1.
- Benign.
- Malignant.
- Inconclusive e.g. cells present but not diagnostic.
- Unsatisfactory/inadequate e.g. minimal or no cells present.

The answer to this is specific to the lesion being biopsied. The result usually comes with a score of 1-5 (e.g. Thy1/Thy2/Thy3 etc. in Thyroid FNAs). As a general key, 1 is insufficient, 2 is benign, 3 is indeterminate (may require repeat) and 4/5 are likely malignant. It is important to know the individual scoring systems for the lesions being investigated.

Q2. What types of thyroid cancer do you know?

A2.
- Follicular (difficult to differentiate benign/malignant on FNA).
- Papillary (can be difficult to exclude depending on stain used).
- Medullary.
- Anaplastic.

FNA is very important in the management of thyroid nodules and expect to know the characteristics of these groups of patients.

Q3. What are the possible complications?

A3.
- Haematoma.
- Infection.
- Needle tract seeding (rare/unproven in thyroid/breast).

Further Reading

- *Cibas E., Ali S. The Bethesda System for Reporting Thyroid Cytopathology – American Journal of Clinical Pathology 2009;132:658-665 – A very good, free and quick article to read.*

Chapter 8   **Lumbar Puncture**

Scenario
You are the oncall surgical trainee in the neurosurgery ward. You have been asked to perform a Lumbar Puncture on a patient with a suspected subarachnoid haemorrhage.

Important points not to miss
As with all the practical scenarios you must interact with the patient in a professional manner and try to put them at ease. This station is about patient safety, applied anatomy and about performing the procedural skill. You must know the contraindications of lumbar puncture, the surface landmarks and the structures that your needle will pass through.

Talk through
Lumbar puncture is commonly performed in neurosurgical units in order to sample CSF and measure intracranial pressure. You may be asked to perform a lumbar puncture on a simulated spine model. You will be marked on obtaining informed consent, undertaking the procedure and in your ability to discuss subsequent patient management.

Indications
- CSF sampling.
- Microscopy and culture.
- Virology.
- CSF protein, biochemistry.

Xanthochromia index (for subarachnoid blood)

- CSF pressure testing.
  ‣ Opening pressure.
  ‣ Pressure reduction by drawing off CSF.
- Spinal anaesthesia.

Contraindications
- Patient refusal.
- Increased intracranial pressure (ICP) as lumbar puncture can result in brainstem herniation.
- As a precaution, CT brain is advocated by some, especially in the following situations.
  ‣ Age >65.
  ‣ Reduced GCS or unconscious state.

- ‣ Recent history of seizure.
- ‣ Focal neurological signs.
- ‣ Ophthalmoscopy for papilledema.

Other contraindications
- Bleeding diathesis.
- Coagulopathy.
- Decreased platelet count (<50 x 10^9/L).
- Infections.
- Skin infection at puncture site.
- Sepsis.
- Abnormal respiratory pattern.
- Hypertension with bradycardia and deteriorating consciousness.
- Vertebral deformities (scoliosis or kyphosis).

Inform patient and consent for
- Post dural puncture headache (1% risk).
- Nerve damage.
- CSF infection/abscess.
- Haematoma formation.
- Persistent CSF leak.
- Failure of procedure.
- Transient paraesthesia.
- Allergic reaction to local anaesthesia.

Equipment
- Sterile gloves and gown.
- Skin preparation solution e.g., chlohexidine, povidone iodine or alcohol.
- Syringes.
- Local anaesthetic e.g. lidocaine 1% 10mls.
- Needles 20G/24G.
- Spinal needle.
- Manometer set.
- Sampling tubes labelled 1,2,3,4.
- Xanthochromia bottle.

Procedure

Sitting, or lateral with hips flexed (sitting usually preferable). Tuffier's line is a line joining the iliac crests at the level of the L3 -4 intervertebral space. Spinous processes of the L3 and 4 vertebrae can be felt in the midpoint either side of this line.

Prepare the skin with aqueous or alcoholic chlorhexidine 2% and allow to dry. Wash your hands after wearing a mask and hat. Using aseptic technique, don your gown and gloves.

Drape the back with sterile drapes.

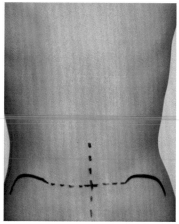

Figure 8.1: Tuffier's Line: A line drawn across the posterior superior iliac crests will intersect the midline at the L3/4 interspace.

After warning patient, infiltrate local anaesthestic passing from the skin to the interspinous ligament or periosteum. Insert the spinal needle with a cranial inclination of 30° at the midpoint between spinous processes, aiming for the umbilicus.

Once through skin, the fat will feel loose. Soon there may be a 'gritty' feeling as the supraspinous ligament is contacted. The interspinous ligament holds the needle firmly but yields with pressure. There may be another 'gritty' feeling as the needle crosses the ligamentum flavum and then a subtle pop as the dura mater is breached. Once in the subarachnoid space, CSF will flow back and drip from the luer of the needle.

At this stage you should offer to measure the opening pressure with the manometer. To do this, you connect the manometer tubing ensuring that the tap valve is open and allow the CSF to rise up the column. It may take some time to reach an equilibrium. Read from the bottom of the meniscus. You may then turn the tap valve to allow the CSF to flow into your waiting sterile containers.

Allow CSF into the containers in order: 1,2,3,4 and finally xanthochromia index. You do not need to fill them. 1ml in each will suffice.

Remove the spinal needle and apply a sterile occlusive dressing.
It is important to nurse patient in supine position for 1 hour post procedure and ensure that they are well hydrated.

Advise staff to contact you or the team if the patient complains of persistent headache or has other pertinent symptoms.

Clearly document procedure in the notes including

- Amount and type of local anaesthetic used.
- Time and date.
- Complications or difficulties encountered, if any.

Sample mark scheme

Introduction, confirms patient identity	0	1	2
Professionalism	0	1	2
Consent (nerve damage, failure etc.)	0	1	2
Positions appropriately	0	1	
Offers to scrub up	0	1	
Prepare and drape area	0	1	
Identifies landmarks (Tuffier's line, midline spinous processes)	0	1	2
Injects local anaesthetic	0	1	
Warns the patient	0	1	
Aims 30° towards umbilicus	0	1	
Explains feeling for two pops	0	1	
Removes stylet	0	1	
Offers to measure opening pressure	0	1	
Takes 3 different samples	0	1	
Offers to label samples 1,2,3,4	0	1	
Sends samples for appropriate investigations	0	1	

FOLLOW ON QUESTIONS

Q1. When is a lumbar puncture contraindicated?

A1. See pages 40 and 41.

Q2. Name the anatomical structures your needle passes through during a lumbar puncture

A2.

- Skin.
- Fat.
- Thoracolumbar fascia.
- Supraspinous ligament.
- Interspinous ligament.
- Ligamentum flavum.
- Epidural fat.
- Dura mater.
- Arachnoid mater.

Q3. Where is CSF produced, where does it travel and how is it absorbed?

A3. The majority of the CSF (60%) is produced in the Choroid Plexus in the lateral ventricles. It circulates from the lateral ventricles via the foramina of Monro to the third ventricle and from there to the fourth ventricle via the aqueduct of Sylvius. It then exits the fourth ventricle via the foramen of Magendie (medially) and foramina of Luschka (Laterally) into the subarachnoid space.

CSF is reabsorbed into venous sinus blood via arachnoid granulations, the largest of which is in the superior sagittal sinus.

Q4. What simultaneous test must you do when doing an LP?

A4. Plasma glucose. CSF should be about 60% of the plasma concentration.

Q5. What causes a post LP headache?

A5. It is widely accepted that a post LP headache occurs due to the stretching and eventual rupture of subdural veins. It is caused by intracranial hypotension from the CSF sampling or an ongoing leak. It typically presents a few days after LP and is made worse by standing. Treatment includes bed rest, hydration and autologous blood patching. It is important not to miss an iatrogenic subdural haemorrhage.

Further Reading

- *National Institute of Clinical Excellence Guidelines. June 2012. Lumbar puncture for suspected bacterial meningitis.*

Chapter 9   Male Urethral Catheterisation

Scenario
You are the urology core trainee who has been called to the Emergency Department. The patient has been assessed by the emergency doctor and has been diagnosed with acute urinary retention. Please insert a urethral catheter.

Important points not to miss
There are a number of ways to insert a urethral catheter, but familiarise yourself with a system that you can use in the exam. This is a very common procedure and, unlike some other procedures, you can practice it a number of times in the wards before the exam. You can use the 'two glove technique' or the 'dirty hand, clean hand' technique, whereby the outside glove it taken off and the inside clean glove is used when touching the catheter. Nonetheless, please practice an aseptic technique you are comfortable with and demonstrate it in the exam.

Talk through
Male catheterisation and issues surrounding this procedure are very common in the exam. You may be asked to talk through and perform the procedure without examining the patient. You will be required to obtain consent and perform the procedure on an actor with an artificial catheterisation system between his legs. Questions will then be centred on problems and complications that you may encounter.

Indications
- Acute urinary retention.
- Chronic urinary retention.
- Frank haematuria to prevent clot retention (3 way catheter).
- Hourly urine output monitoring in an unwell patient.
- Peri-operative (pelvic access/prolonged procedure).
- Urinary incontinence (relative indication).

Contraindication
- Urethral Injury following pelvic trauma.

Consent
It is not necessary to obtain written consent for catheterisation.
- Talk through the procedure in layman's terms.

- Indication for procedure.
- Risks, if not performed.
- Alternatives.
- What the procedure entiles.
- Complications.
  - Failure (need for alternatives).
  - False passage.
  - Haematuria.
  - Pain (bladder spasm).
- Occasional need for monitoring urine output post catheterisation (diuresis).

Equipment
A second examiner may act as an assistant and offer to get a trolley ready for you.
- Basic catheter pack.
  - Kidney dish, gallipot, gauze and sterile drape.
- Skin preparation solution (sterile water is acceptable).
- Sterile gloves.
- Appropriate urinary catheter (14 Ch is probably the most appropriate; ensure that it is not a female catheter as these are shorter).
- 10ml syringe + 10ml water (not saline) if not supplied with catheter.
- Instillagel (anaesthetic, antiseptic lubricant) – minimum 10ml.
- Appropriate catheter bag (large 'night' bag or a urometer).

Positioning
Patient should be as flat as possible to perform the procedure. Attempt to reassure them and talk through the procedure to prevent the patient from sitting up to see what is going on. Ensure the patient is exposed at the latest possible moment and covered as soon as possible. The procedure can be embarrassing and has a significant impact on a patient's self image. Exposure should be from xiphisternum to knees.

Procedure
The following is based around the guidelines from the European Association of Urological Nurses.

Confirm patient's identity and ask if they have previously had a catheter and, if so, whether any problem or complications were encountered. Ask for allergies (iodine/chlorhexidine/lignocaine/latex) before positioning the patient supine and covering them. Wash your hands and prepare your equipment. Ask the assistant to obtain adequate exposure. Cleanse hands with an alcohol-based agent and don non-sterile gloves.

Use one hand to retract the foreskin with gauze and clean the foreskin, glans and meatus (separate swabs for each). Change to sterile gloves and apply a sterile drape. Place the kidney dish or collecting dish between the patient's legs. Instil at least 10ml of gel into the urethra, hold the urethra at the base of the glans and wait for 3-5 minutes.

Advance the catheter with the penis held pointing to the ceiling with gentle traction. Pass the catheter all the way to the hilt and wait for urine to drain.

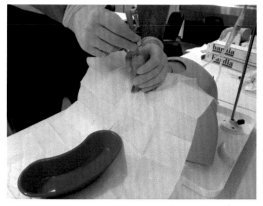

After urine has started to drain, inflate the balloon with the appropriate amount of sterile water (usually 10mL, but some such as 3-way catheters require 30mL) and withdraw the catheter gently. Replace the foreskin if present. Dry and cover the patient before asking them to redress. Dispose off the

Figure 9.1: Catheter insertion: Hold the penis pointing directly upwards and pass the catheter in to the hilt.

equipment in the appropriate bin. Measure the amount of urine draining after an adequate period of time (5-10 minutes) and obtain a CSU for microscopy, culture and sensitivity.

Document the procedure in the notes:
- Date and time.
- Indication.
- Consent obtained.
- Size and type of catheter (use sticker if available).
- Complications/Difficulties if any.
- Volume used to inflate balloon.
- Colour of urine +/- presence of sediment.
- Residual volume in bladder.
- Date required for change if a long-term device.

Sample mark scheme

Introduction and consent	0	1	2
Professionalism	0	1	2
Checks allergies and previous complications	0	1	2
Positions patient appropriately and adequate exposure	0	1	
Checks catheter type and expiry date	0	1	
Opens catheter pack using aseptic technique	0	1	
Cleans meatus and glans	0	1	
Changes to sterile gloves	0	1	
Instils local anaesthetic gel and holds for 3 minutes	0	1	
Passes catheter while maintaining aseptic technique	0	1	
Drains urine before inflating balloon with 10ml water	0	1	
Communicates with patient throughout the procedure	0	1	
Attaches catheter bag	0	1	
Repositions foreskin (if present)	0	1	
Covers patient	0	1	
Documents the procedure in the notes appropriately	0	1	2

FOLLOW ON QUESTIONS

Q1. What would you do if no urine drains after catheterisation?

A1.

- Reevaluate presence of urine in bladder by percussing the suprapubic region if you haven't done this already. Apply suprapubic pressure.
- Aspirate with a syringe.
- Flush with a 50ml catheter syringe and sterile water.

Q2. What are the complications of urinary catheterisation?

A2. See page 47

Q3. At what volume would you consider a patient to be in retention?

A3. Five hundred milliliters is the typical quoted value for acute urinary retention in an otherwise normal bladder, but this can change significantly in pathological processes (shrunken bladders/chronic urinary retention)

Q4. What options can you consider if you fail to insert a urethral catheter?

A4.

- Try a larger stiffer catheter such as silicone catheter.
- Consider using a coudé tip in patients with large prostates.
- Supra-pubic catheter.
- Urethral catheter under flexible-cystoscopic guidance.
- Use of 'specialist' catheters/introducer.

If you do not know how to do any of the above, state that you would discuss the case with a senior urologist on-call, but are aware of these options.

Q5. What are the causes of renal failure?

A5. It is important to divide your answer into pre-renal, intrinsic and post renal causes.

Prerenal - renal hypoperfusion due to hypovolemia; Volume overload with reduced renal perfusion as in severe congestive heart failure; Peripheral vasodilation as in septic shock.

Intrinsic - associated with ATN following severe systemic insult, e.g., surgery, trauma, burns, hypotension and sepsis; Acute interstitial nephritis; Atheroembolic acute kidney injury following vascular procedures or contrast studies; Nephrotoxic drugs such as aminoglycosides.

Postrenal - caused by urinary tract obstruction. Ureteric obstruction (e.g., tumours, stones, fibrosis); Bladder outflow obstruction (e.g., prostatism)

Q6. What types of catheters do you know?

A6.
- Short-term (yellow/orange) vs. Long-term (grey).
- Latex (normal) vs. Non-latex (silicone).
- 1-way (for intermittent catheterisation), 2-way (normal) and 3-way (for irrigation).
- Balloon size – 10 ml (normal) 30-50ml (post prostatectomy for haemostasis).
- Specialist catheters – Silver tip (reduce infection), coudé (curved) tipped.

Q7. You insert the catheter; it drains no urine and you therefore remove it. You then examine this patient's abdomen and there is a supra-pubic mass. What is your differential diagnosis?

A7.
- A bladder that was not catheterised appropriately.
- Colonic carcinoma.
- Large iliac aneurysm.

This is a very unusual question but can be asked. The aorta bifurcates at the level of the umbilicus (lower border of L4 vertebra) and it is therefore unlikely to be an aortic aneurysm. The iliac vessels lie in the hypogastric (suprapubic) region.

Further Reading

- *Evidence-based Guidelines for Best Practice in Urological Health Care: Catheterisation Indwelling catheters in adults - Urethral and Suprapubic - European Association of Urology Nurses (a comprehensive, free, online guidance)*

Chapter	10	**Organising a Theatre List**

Scenario
You can be provided with a list of patients awaiting theatre and asked to write out a theatre list in the most appropriate order. Follow on questions can be about perioperative care and surgical safety.

Examples of patients may include:
- Incarcerated hernia in diabetic patient.
    - Diabetic.
    - Emergency.
- Open cholecystectomy in patient with a pacemaker.
    - A pacemaker doesn't dictate order but requires bipolar diathermy.
- Sigmoid colectomy in a patient with MRSA.
    - Patients with infections go last in the list.
    - Clean - Contaminated procedure.

Important things not to miss
There may be more than one correct list order but it is important to be able to justify your decision to the examiner. It is also important to write legibly and fill in details that the anaesthetist may want such as medical co-morbidities and coagulopathies as well as the important surgical details such as laterality. Don't forget to sign, date and add the time to the bottom of the hand written list.

Talk through
- Patients with diabetes go early in the list.
This prevents complications of hypoglycaemia and allows early return to normal glycaemic control. Peri and post-operative normoglycaemia is essential in order to reduce rates of surgical site infections.
- Patients with latex allergies should be considered to be first in the list.
Natural rubber allergies require a clean theatre and time must be given for previous latex "dust" to settle before starting the case. All latex products must be removed form theatre or clearly labelled. Latex products like catheters must also be removed. Latex products can be removed the day before if the list is scheduled.
- Children should be operated on early.
This minimises distress to the child and the parents.
- Procedure under local anaesthesia (minor point)

Some surgeons would put local anaesthetic cases first or last as a professional courtesy to their anaesthetic colleagues. However, it is also practical to place small local anaesthetic cases between major cases to allow the anaesthetist to recover the last patient and anaesthetise the next to optimise theatre time.

- Major procedures should be considered to be early in the list.

Major procedures and patients for cancer resection should not be cancelled due to time constraints. It is often best to put these cases first or early on the list.

- Patients with infection go last in the list.

MRSA and C.*difficile* must go last on a list to prevent cross contamination between patients. If possible, order a list according to USA NRCS guidelines (Clean, Clean-contaminated, Contaminated, Dirty). See chapter 15, page 84".

- Clinical Priority.

It is important to appreciate the difference in operative priority between emergency and elective procedures. Life- or limb-threatening conditions must go first on an emergency list. Please learn the National Confidential Enquiry into Patient Outcome and Death (NCEPOD) Criteria for emergency surgery since you maybe asked to give examples.

1a. Immediate.
- Life or limb threatening.
- Simultaneous haemodynamic resuscitation and intervention.
- Ruptured AAA, Ruptured spleen and Haemodynamically unstable pelvic trauma.

1b. < 6 hours.
- Life threatening but not immediate.
- Intervention following resuscitation.
- Ischaemic bowel, large bowel obstruction.

2. <24 hours.
- Urgent.
- Deterioration of condition that may threaten life.
- Appendicitis (not perforated).

3. < 7 days.
- Deterioration of elective condition.
- Acute cholecystectomy.

4. Scheduled.
- Elective procedure with no threat to life or limb.

Sample mark scheme

Legible documentation	0	1	
Correct theatre/staff details	0	1	
Correct patient details	0	1	2
Correct operation details	0	1	2
Acceptable order for theatre list	0	1	
List signed/dated	0	1	2
Awareness of NCEPOD and examples	0	1	2
Understands peri-operative glycaemic control	0	1	2
Awareness of critical patients (infections/latex allergy)	0	1	2
Aware of minor considerations for listing (local anaesthetic/day case/children)	0	1	
Understands peri-operative risks for wound infection	0	1	2
Able to discuss and rationalise use antibiotic prophylaxis	0	1	
Understands peri-operative management of implantable devices	0	1	

FOLLOW ON QUESTIONS

Q1. What perioperative measure can reduce surgical site infection rates?

A1.
- Tight glycaemic control.
- Oxygen supplementation.
- Maintain normothermia.
- Careful preparation and draping.

Note: There is no evidence to suggest that laminar flow or space suits reduce infection rates.

Q2. When are prophylactic antibiotics indicated in surgery?

A2.
- When the risk of infection is high (>4%).
  ‣ Clean-contaminated "single dose".
  ‣ Contaminated "3 doses".
  ‣ Dirty "Prolonged".
- High Risk Patient factors.
  ‣ Immunocompromise.
  ‣ Poorly controlled diabetes.
  ‣ Malnutrition.
  ‣ High Body Mass index.
- High risk procedures.
  ‣ Orthopaedic or Vascular Implant surgery.
  ‣ Entry into Bone Cavities e.g. Sternotomy.
  ‣ Metallic or other prosthetic heart valves.

Q3. What are the current guidelines for perioperative glycaemic control in the diabetic patient?

A3.
- Patients with diabetes must be prioritised in the operating list.
- Routine overnight admission is not necessary.
- Starvation time should be no more than one missed meal.
- Analgesia and anti-emetics should be used to enable early return to diet and usual insulin regime.
- Insulin infusions should only be used if a patient is expected to miss more than one meal.
- 0.45% sodium chloride with 5% glucose and 0.15% or 0.3% KCl is the recommended IV fluid.

- Capillary blood glucose should be measure hourly during and after the any surgical procedure.
- The WHO surgical safety checklist should identify all diabetic patients.
- The target blood glucose should be 6-10 mmol/L (acceptable range 4-12 mmol/L).

Note: The term "sliding scale" is now replaced with the term "variable rate intra-venous insulin".

Q4. What are the guidelines for patients with continuous subcutaneous insulin infusions (CSII)?

A4.
There are no specific guidelines at present for this situation. Some anaesthetists will allow the use of a CSII before and during the procedure providing they have checked that the pump is working, it has been placed away from the surgical field for 24 hours and blood glucose can be measured every hour. If the anaesthetist is not happy to use a CSII or any of the above conditions are not met, they will use an alternative method of glycaemic control such as a variable rate intravenous infusion.

Q5. When should metformin be stopped before an operation?

A5. There is currently no consensus but the majority of anaesthetists suggest omitting metformin on the morning of the procedure to reduce the possibility of lactic acidosis and renal impairment. It is also suggested by the Royal College of Radiologists that any patient receiving intravenous or intra-arterial iodinated contrast with an eGFR < 60ml/min should omit their metformin for 48 hours post procedure.

Further Reading

- *National Enquiry into Patient Outcome and Death 2011.*
- *Management of adults with diabetes undergoing surgery and elective procedures: improving standards. NHS Diabetes 2012.*

Chapter 11 — Theatre Safety and design

Scenarios
Although not a station in itself, you may be asked specific questions about theatre safety after the "organising a theatre list", "removal of a naevus" and "surgical scrubbing" stations.

1. What systems are in place to ensure patient safety and reduce avoidable errors in theatre?

2. Having scrubbed and gowned you are asked to perform the WHO check list. What does this involve?

3. What perioperative interventions reduce the possibility of surgical infections?

4. How is an operating theatre laid out? How does this help reduce infections?

Important points not to miss
You must be able to list the three components of the WHO checklist and explain what each component entails. It will become clear that you have not been part of a theatre team if you cannot do so. It is also essential that you can explain some of the steps taken to minimise surgical site infections. Most candidates simply say antiseptic preparations, gloves, gowns and antibiotics. As with all questions in surgery you must classify your answer, for example: "There are steps that can be taken in the pre-operative, intra-operative and post-operative periods to reduce surgical infections".

Pre-operative interventions include chlorhexadine showering, hair removal on surgical site using a single use electric razor on the day of surgery, and theatre staff removing hand jewellery.

Intraoperative methods to reduce infection include; antibiotic prophylaxis if appropriate, maintaining patient normothermia and glycaemia hand decontamination; sterile gowns for theatre staff; skin preparation and draping of patient in a well-ventilated theatre.

Postoperative methods include aseptic dressings for wounds, wound care advice to patient and appropriate ward care by staff with regular review.

Theatre design can be explained using basic principles. Operating theatres should be located near to related facilities, for example, Accident and Emergency, Radiology and Intensive Care. Theatres should also away from main entrances and public areas. Theatres themselves should be big enough to hold the required staff and equipment necessary together with the patient. The theatre is focused around the operating table, with access required to it from the anaesthetic room, scrub room, preparation room and recovery area. The theatre should also have easy access to control the temperature, humidity, ventilation and light.

Talk through

The world health organization has undertaken a number of initiatives to address surgical safety. The world alliance for patient safety started in 2007 and focused on the WHO safe surgery checklist. The checklist highlights three phases during surgery. These are the sign in-pre induction of anaesthesia, sign out-pre incision of skin, and sign out-pre transfer of patient from theatre.

All members of the theatre staff are involved, anaesthetic nurses and staff, along with theatre staff are involved in the initial sign in, the anaesthetic staff then hand over the anaesthetised patient into theatre during the first sign out, with the theatre staff signing the patient out prior to transfer to recovery

Sign in (before induction of anaesthesia)
- Patient has confirmed:
  ‣ Identity.
  ‣ Site.
  ‣ Procedure.
  ‣ Consent.
- Site marked (if applicable).
- Anaesthesia safety check confirmed.
- Confirm any allergy.
- Airway and bleeding risks highlighted and appropriate precaution taken (difficult airway trolley, aspiration risk, group and save, adequate intravenous access and fluids planned).

Time out (before skin incision)
- Introduce all members of the team and their roles.
- Confirm patient name, site and procedure.
- Confirm instrument sterility.
- Surgeons highlight any anticipated critical events- e.g., blood loss.
- Anaesthetic team highlight any patient specific concerns (glycaemia control, cardiac risks, problems at induction).
- Antibiotic prophylaxis given/needed within last 60 mins.
- Thromoboprophlaxis given/needed.
- Essential imaging displayed.

Sign out (before patient leaves operating room)
- Confirm name and site of procedure.
- Confirm swab and instrument count correct.
- Confirm specimens are labeled (if appropriate).
- Any equipment problems.
- Any concerns to be handed over to recovery staff?

This may be more depth than you will need for the exam but a decent knowledge of the process is not only good practice but repeatedly comes up in various aspects of the exam.

Mark scheme

Confirms name and details of patient pre op	0	1	
Confirms procedure and that site is marked	0	1	
Able to highlight potential intra operative risks	0	1	2
Understands reasons for use of WHO checklist	0	1	
Provides 2 components of WHO sign in	0	1	2
Provides 2 components of WHO sign out	0	1	2
Able to formulate a post op plan, awareness of risks	0	1	2
Provides two or more other methods for reducing operative risk	0	1	2
Awareness of when WHO checklist takes place	0	1	
Understands members of team involved in WHO checklist	0	1	

FOLLOW ON QUESTIONS

Q1. What other measures do you know to improve operative safety?

A1.
- Surgical measures - appropriate experience/supervision, communication in theatre, anticipating events and planning for them, e.g., bleeding - ensuring cross - matched blood is available.
- Environmental - calming/quiet atmosphere, quiet music, theatre design and layout, appropriate monitoring.
- Others - specialist teams, pre op assessment, regular auditing of results, adequate staffing, patient identification bands.

Q2. What patient factors can be manipulated to reduce the risk of infection?

A2.
- Short pre operative stay.
- Shave patient in theatre prior to surgery.
- Remove ward blankets and clothing before entering theatre.

Q3. How can the lay out of a theatre complex affect patient safety?

A3.
- ITU nearby and on same level.
- Close proximity to emergency and radiology departments.
- Away from main entrance and general hospital traffic.
- Theatres should be next to each other to reduce staff movement.
- Anaesthetic rooms should be adjacent to theatres.
- Sterile services in the unit.

Q4. Describe how you would prepare the patients skin prior to surgery?

A4.
- Operation site should be removed of hair in theatre.
- Operation site and surrounding area should be cleaned using a sponge or swab impregnated with detergent.
- Skin is prepared with alcohol based chlorhexidine or povidone-iodine. This should be dried completely and should not pool.
- Skin should be prepared from the cleanest area to the dirtiest area.

Q5. What are the criteria for consideration of day surgery?

A5.
- Patients must be ASA I or II.
- BMI < 35.
- Projected operation time of < 1 hour.
- Must be acceptable to patient.
- Must have home support on discharge and a home phone.
- Must live close to the hospital.

Q6. How are patients stratified for risk of DVT?

A6.
Patients are stratified according to their pre operative condition, risk factors, and type of operation

Low risk-
- Minor surgery-(<30min) no other risk factors besides age.
- Major surgery- (>30min) <40 years of age with no other risk factors.
- Minor trauma or medical illness.

Moderate risk-
- Major general, urological, gynaecological surgery plus age of >40.
- Major medical illness or malignancy.
- Major trauma or burns.
- Minor surgery with previous DVT/PE or thrombophilia.

High risk -
- Facture or major orthopaedic surgery of pelvis/hips/lower limb.
- Major pelvic or abdominal surgery for neoplasia.
- Major surgery or illness with previous DVT/PE/proven thrombophilia.
- Major lower limb amputation.

Chapter	12	**Removal of a Naevus**

Scenario

You are doing a day case list with your consultant and the next case is an excision biopsy of a naevus. Your consultant has been called away to an emergency and you have been asked to continue with the operation. The patient has been consented and local anaesthetic has already been infiltrated.

Important points not to miss

You will be making a mistake if you rush to excise the naevus since you will miss vital marks prior to the procedure being carried out. As in all stations in the exam, read the scenario carefully to understand exactly what your task is. When entering the room, use the alcohol gel provided and introduce yourself to the patient. In this scenario, it would be prudent to briefly explain that the consultant has had to leave due to an emergency and that you will be performing the procedure.

Talk through

This is a common station in the exam and you should be comfortable in undertaking this task. The scenario might state that the consultant has administered the local anaesthetic prior to leaving for an emergency. You will be expected to gather the appropriate equipment, undertake the procedure and then answer relevant follow on questions. The examiner may play the part of the patient and the naevus might be on a foam pad (similar to those found in most clinical skills labs).

Consent & mark

Although the scenario states the patient has already been consented, as the operating surgeon, you must check the consent form yourself:

- Is this the correct patient (triple identification)?
- Is it the correct procedure?
- Is it the correct site and does this correspond to a mark on the patient?
- Has the form been signed by the patient?

Important questions to ask

Before starting your procedure there are a few important things to ask the patient which will likely score you more points.

- Allergies.
- Anticoagulants (Warfarin/Aspirin/Clopidogrel).

- Bleeding disorders.

Equipment

You may be asked to select appropriate equipment from a selection and place a blade on a scalpel using a haemostatic clamp. Therefore, practise this before your exam. However due to time restraints, the correct equipment may be provided for you and the patient already prepared and draped. You will be expected to know which suture is appropriate to use?

- Sterile gloves.
- Sterile pen and ruler.
- Scalpel and no. 10 / 15 blade.
- Toothed forceps.
- Marker stitch.
- Skin suture.
- Adherent dressing.

Marking your incision

If a sterile pen and ruler are available, you should draw out your incision. For an excision biopsy of a naevus, only a small margin is required (2mm). Remember it is a biopsy, you are not performing a wider excision to gain adequate clearance. The wider your excision margin, the more difficult it will be to close the defect! Mark a 2mm margin around the naevus, and extend this into an ellipse with a 3:1 length to width ratio. Ensuring a 3:1 ratio will help to reduce the tension across the defect, making closure easier, and will also help to prevent dog-ears at either end of the wound.

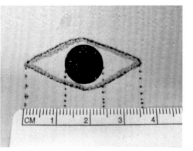

Figure 12.1: *Mark out the naevus: The ellipse length should be three times the width of the lesion.*

Excision

Once you have marked out your incision, before you put blade to skin you must check and ensure that the local anaesthetic has worked. Do this by either pinching the skin gently with toothed forceps or gently testing the skin with the tip of the blade. Excise the naevus along your lines in two continuous strokes of each side, rather than multiple smaller strokes, ensuring to keep the blade perpendicular to the skin. Then using your toothed forceps, pick up one corner and slowly continue to excise the naevus from one end to the other, ensuring to remove a cuff of subcutaneous tissue (sponge) with the naevus. At this point you should offer to mark the sample with a marker stitch for histology. Most commonly this is done with a 3.0 silk suture, placed at a named point on the sample e.g. superior, 12 0'clock. It is important to offer to fill out a histology form with the appropriate clinical information and the marker stitch position documented.

Closure
For the purpose of the exam, close the wound with simple interrupted sutures, using a non-absorbable, monofilament material, such as nylon. The size of the suture used and the length of time they are left in will be determined by the anatomical location of the wound.

Anatomic location	Suture size	When sutures should be removed
Face	5.0 / 6.0	3 - 5 days
Scalp	3.0 / 4.0	5 - 7 days
Limbs	4.0	7-10 days
Back	3.0 / 4.0	10-14 days

Table 12.1: Suture sizes and duration for different anatomical locations

Place an interrupted suture in the centre of the wound to split it into two halves, then place further sutures centrally into each of the 2 halves, and so on. This ensures that the sutures are equally spaced and makes the finished wound appear much neater (which the examiners will notice). Finish by applying a simple adherent dressing to the wound.

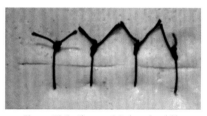

Figure 12.2: Closure: Stitches should be placed with uniform spacing

Post-operative instructions & follow up
Once you have finished the procedure, the first thing you should do is discard your sharps into a sharps bin, which will be provided in the station. At this point, the patient may ask you a few questions regarding post-op instructions, but you will appear far more professional if you offer this information without being prompted. Explain that the patient will go home with some simple analgesia, and that they must seek medical attention if there are any worrying signs/symptoms (increased pain, redness, discharge/blood through dressing etc). Give the patient

the appropriate follow-up information with regards to when and where the sutures must be removed, and that a further clinic appointment will be posted to them once the results are available from histology.

Sample mark scheme

Introduction	0	1	
Checks consent	0	1	2
Checks mark	0	1	
Checks for allergies/Bleeding disorders	0	1	2
Checks local anaesthetic is working	0	1	
Chooses appropriate equipment	0	1	2
Marks elliptical incision (3:1)	0	1	
Removes naevus	0	1	
Closes wound appropriately	0	1	2
Offers to mark the naevus with sutures	0	1	2
Sends for histology	0	1	
Applies appropriate dressing	0	1	
Post op instructions given clearly	0	1	2
Disposes off equipment safely	0	1	

FOLLOW ON QUESTIONS

Q1. How long do you leave sutures in?

A1. Please see table 12.1.

Q2. What are Langer's lines/ Relaxed Skin Tension Lines?

A2. Langer's lines were described by Karl Langer back in the 1860's. Langer used conical spikes to produce multiple elliptical shaped wounds in the skin of cadavers. He made the wounds as close as possible, and when grouped together, they formed the appearance of lines – what we now call 'Langer's lines'. It was only in 1911 that Kocher noted that the appearance of operation scars is greatly improved if the incision is made in the direction of Langer's lines. However, in more recent years, Langer's lines have fallen out of practice and it is now Relaxed Skin Tension Lines (RSTLs) that we use to determine the orientation of our incisions. RSTLs are the tension lines that match the furrows formed in relaxed skin (formed from pinching the skin) and tend to lie perpendicular to the direction of the underlying muscle fibres.

Q3. What is your understanding of Breslow thickness / Clark's Levels in relation to Melanoma?

A3. Breslow thickness is very important in the management of Melanoma, as it not only offers information on prognosis, but it determines further management with regard to wider excision margins. It is the distance between the granular layer of the epidermis and the deepest part of the Melanoma.

Breslow Thickness	Excision margins	Approximate 5 year survival
<1 mm	1cm	95-100%
1 - 2 mm	1-2cm	80-96%
2.1 - 4 mm	2-3cm	60-75%
>4 mm	3cm	50%

Table 12.2: Excision margins at different Breslow thickness and approximate 5 year survival

Clarks five anatomical levels:

1. Melanoma confined to the epidermis (melanoma in situ).
2. Invasion into the papillary dermis.
3. Invasion to the junction of the papillary and reticular dermis.

4. Invasion into the reticular dermis.
5. Invasion into the subcutaneous fat.

Higher the Clark's level, worse the prognosis. However, Clark's level can vary in different anatomical sites and thus they are less reliable in calculating prognosis. They also have a lower predictive value, is less reproducible and more subjective than Breslow depth. (Hence Breslow thickness is widely used in clinical practice in the management of patients and to predict prognosis).

Further Reading

- *Royal College of Surgeons of England Basic Surgical skills Course manual 2007.*
- *British Association of Dermatologists – Guidelines for the management of melanoma.*

Chapter 13 Safe use of Local Anaesthetics

Scenario

This might not be an independent station but questions on local anaesthesia may be asked in the "Removal of a Naevus", "Suturing skills: Closure of a wound" stations. It can also be tested in the Applied Surgical Sciences and Critical Care OSCE stations.

Important points not to miss

The knowledge examined in this station is very important and clinically relevant. Ensure that you are aware of the anatomical sites (e.g., digits, ears and penis) where usage of adrenaline mixed with a local anaesthetic agent is contra--indicated. You should also be familiar with local anaesthetic toxicity as well as the management in case of a reaction.

Talk through

Use of local anaesthetic agents is seen as a core knowledge area. You should have a sound understanding of its mechanism of action, duration of action, safe dosages of commonly used agents, and indications and contraindications for usage of local anaesthesia.

Local anaesthetics are water soluble drugs that cause temporary (reversible) anaesthesia and loss of nociception. They are often combined with vasoconstrictive additives such as adrenaline and synthetic vasopressin in order to reduce the rate of absorption and prolong the duration of action.

Local anaesthetics are used for
- Superficial surgical procedures.
- Regional anaesthetic blocks (nerve and plexus).
- Central neuraxial techniques such as spinal or epidural block.
- IV regional anaesthesia (Bier's block).
- Post operative pain relief via infiltration or catheter techniques.

All local anaesthetics contain a lipophilic aromatic group and a hydrophilic group. These two structures are linked by either an amide or ester group. Amide anaesthetics are stable and have a long shelf life while esters are more volatile and unstable in solution. It is important to know a few examples of each.

Amides
- Lidocaine (lignocaine Xylocaine®).
- Bupivacaine (Marcaine®, Chirocaine®).

Esters
- Cocaine.
- Amethocaine.

Additives
- Adrenaline 1:200,000.

Local anaesthetics act by blocking the Na+ channel within the nerve. The lipid soluble drug passes through the cell membrane where it becomes ionized. It is then able to bind to the inner surface of the sodium channel, preventing it from activating. The potency of a local anaesthetic is therefore directly related to the dose and the lipid solubility.

It is essential that you know the maximum safe dose of local anaesthetics. Lidocaine and bupivocaine are the most commonly used local anaesthetics in general surgical practice. The maximum safe dose of lidocaine is 3mg/kg without adrenaline but up to 7mg/kg can be given with adrenaline. Because adrenaline is a vasoconstrictor it reduces the amount of vascular "wash out" and it is therefore safe to use a higher dose of lidocaine. Bupivacaine is more cardiotoxic than lidocaine because it is more lipid soluble. The maximum safe dose of bupivacaine is therefore 2mg/kg with or without adrenaline.

In order to calculate the maximum amount of local anaesthetic, one must understand that 100% concentration is 1g (or 1,000mg) per ml. Therefore, 10% concentration is 100mg per ml and 1% is 10mg per ml.

For example, if you wish to administer a 60kg woman the maximum safe dose of 1% plain lidocaine, please bear in mind that the maximum dose of lidocaine without adrenaline is 3mg/kg. Therefore, the maximum safe dose will be 60kg x 3mg/kg = 180mg. In order to work out the volume you can infiltrate, remember that 1% solution is equivalent to 10mg per ml (100% is 1,000mg/ml). Thus the maximum safe dose divided by the concentration will give you the safe volume for infiltration. In this instance, it is 180mg / 10mg per ml = **18 ml**. If it is 2% plain lidocaine (20mg per ml), then the maximum safe dose will be 180mg / 20mg per ml = 9ml.

If the drug is 1% lidocaine with adrenaline, then the maximum safe dose is 5-7 mg/kg. For the purpose of this discussion, if we calculate it as 5 mg/kg, then the maximum safe dose will be 60kg x 5mg/kg = 300mg, which is equivalent to **30 ml** (300mg / 10mg per ml).

Patients who receive more than the safe dose of local anaesthetic may not display signs of toxicity immediately. Any patient who has received local anaesthetic and develops an altered mental state or becomes agitated must be assumed to have exceeded the safe dosage. The classic signs are disinhibition and peri oral tingling. They may develop cardiovascular symptoms such as sinus bradycardia, conduction blocks, asystole or ventricular tachyarrhythmias. Treatment is supportive with airway control, ventilation and circulatory support. The local anaesthetic injection should be immediately stopped and a bolus of 20% lipid emulsion given (1.5ml/kg over 1 minute). Further boluses can be given up to a maximum of 12ml/kg.

Sample mark scheme

Aware of indications of use of local anaesthetics	0	1	2
Aware of classes of local anaesthetics	0	1	2
Understands mechanism of action of local anaesthetic	0	1	2
Able to name three local anaesthetics (all 3 for 2 marks)	0	1	2
Able to name one long-acting local anaesthetic	0	1	
Aware of additives (adrenaline)	0	1	
Safe dose of Lignocaine			
‣ Without adrenaline.	0	1	
‣ With adrenaline.	0	1	
Able to calculate appropriate maximum dose	0	1	2
Aware of complications of local anaesthetic	0	1	2
Aware of presenting symptoms of toxicity	0	1	2
Able to state safe management of local anaesthetic toxicity	0	1	2

FOLLOW ON QUESTIONS

Q1. What is the maximum safe dose of local anaesthetic?

A1.
- Lidocaine – 3mg/kg (5-7mg/kg with 1:200,000 adrenaline).
- Bupivacaine – 2mg/kg (with or without adrenaline).

Q2. You wish to give a 70kg man 0.5% bupivacaine in his post operative wound. He has received no local anaesthetics so far. How much can you give him?

A2.
Concentrations
- 0.25% = 2.5mg/ml.
- 0.5% = 5mg/ml.
- 1% = 10mg/ml.
- 2% = 20mg/ml.

So maximum volume of 0.5% bupivacaine in a 70kg man is:

Weight x Safe dose
70(kg) x 2(mg/kg) =140mg
0.5% = 5mg/ml
140/5 = 28mls

Q3. What influences the potency of an anaesthetic?

A3. Potency depends on the dose and lipid solubility.

Q4. What influence the duration of action of a local anaesthetic?

A4. Duration of action is related to the degree of protein binding. Vascularity of the area treated is also a factor with high blood flow causing "Washing out" of the agent.

Q5. What influences the cardiotoxicity of a local anaesthetic?

A5. Lidocaine is less lipid soluble and has less protein binding than Bupivacaine. Thus Lidocaine is less cardiotoxic than Bupivacaine.

Q6. Why do certain local anaesthetics have a quicker onset than others?

A6. This depends on the pKa (amount of unionized vs ionized drug at a certain pH). Unionized drug can cross lipid bilayers more rapidly. Lidocaine is more unionized at physiological pH than Bupivacaine, hence more rapid onset.

Q7. What is the mechanism of action of local anaesthetics?

A7. Local anaesthetics block the sodium channel in nerve axons, preventing depolarization, thus causing interruption in neuronal transmission.

Q8. How would local anaesthetic toxicity present?

A8.
- Circumoral tingling and paraesthesia.
- Disinhibition.
- Fitting.
- Depression of consciousness.
- Coma.
- Cardiac disturbances e.g. ventricular fibrillation or torsade du points.

Q9. What is the treatment of local anaesthetic toxicity?

A9.
- Stop administering the local anaesthetic.
- Call for help.
- 100% oxygen.
- ABC approach – may require intubation or ventilatory support.
- Efforts of CPR for loss of cardiac output may be prolonged for up to an hour.
- Bolus of 20% lipid emulsion (1.5ml/kg over 1 minute) to bind the remaining local anaesthetic. Commonly used drug is Intralipid©.

Further Reading

- *Management of Severe Local Anaesthetic Toxicity. The Association of Anaesthetists of Great Britain & Ireland 2010.*

| Chapter | 14 | **Scrubbing up for Theatre** |

Scenario
You have been asked to assist your Consultant in performing a hip hemiarthroplasty. Please prepare yourself to join him at the operating table.

Important points not to miss
This is a very common station and at first glance looks very simple but under the pressure of the exam it is easy to miss important steps. It is essential that you do not miss important steps such as brushing your fingernails or wearing a hat. You are most likely to complete this station in time to answer the follow on questions.

Talk through
Preparation
First, offer to change into theatre attire including clogs (although the examiner might not ask you to do). Then find a theatre cap and mask. You must wear some form of eye protection. This might be specific surgical glasses or a visor on the mask. If a mask with eye protection is available you should wear this one. It is unlikely that you will be asked to scrub for a procedure using fluoroscopy but read the question carefully as you may need to wear a lead gown. Remove all jewellery except a plain wedding band which is permitted. Surgeons should not wear false nails, nail varnish or polish. Offer to remove these if you have forgotten on the day.

Scrubbing
An eight stage hand washing process is currently recommended by the Association for Perioperative Practice 2007 (modified from the Ayliffe's six step technique). Each stage involves 5 strokes rubbing the hands backwards and forwards. At every stage you must keep your hands above your elbows to ensure no water runs from an unclean area to your clean hands.

Pre wash
- Open Scrub brush/nail pick packet.
- Wash hands with running water and approximately 5mls antimicrobial solution.
- Remove debris from under nails using a nail pick.
- Rinse hands.

Hand Wash
- Apply surgical scrub to palms.

- Rotate hands and move one hand up the arm to the elbow.
- Repeat on other side.
- Interlace fingers - Right over left along the length of the fingers.
- Then Left over Right.
- Palm to Palm.
- Clasp your thumb in your palm and rotate.
- Clasp your hands together so the dorsal aspects of the interphalangeal joints are in contact with the contralateral palm.

Scrub brush
- Remove scrub brush from packet.
- Add approximately 5mls of antimicrobial solution to moist brush.
- Scrub finger nails & cuticles. Use sponge on finger web spaces.
- Discard brush and rinse hands.

Hand Wash
- Apply surgical scrub to palms.
- Rotate hands and move one hand up the arm to the elbow.
- Repeat on other side.
- Interlace fingers - Right over left along the length of the fingers.
- Then Left over Right.
- Palm to Palm.
- Clasp your thumb in your palm and rotate.
- Clasp your hands together so the dorsal aspects of the interphalangeal joints are in contact with the contralateral palm.

Rotation
- Apply surgical scrub to palms.
- Rotate hands and move one hand up the arm to 2 fingers width above the elbow.
- Repeat on other side.
- Rinse with water – always from hand to elbow.

Hand Wash
- Apply surgical scrub to palms.
- Rotate hands and move one hand up the arm to the elbow.
- Repeat on other side.
- Interlace fingers - Right over left along the length of the fingers.
- Then Left over Right.
- Palm to Palm.
- Clasp your thumb in your palm and rotate.
- Clasp your hands together so the dorsal aspects of the interphalangeal joints are in contact with the contralateral palm.

Drying
- With one towel in the palm of one hand dry from hand to elbow of opposite hand.
- Discard towel.
- Repeat on other side.

Gowning and Gloving

The outer wrap of the gown pack is opened by a Nurse, Health Care Assistant (HCA) or Operation Department Practitioner (ODP). The Inner wrap is opened by the Surgeon. Only touch the inside/spine of the garment and locate the sleeve openings. Check there is nothing next to you that might contaminate you. Open, (not shake) the gown and push your arms into the sleeves, keeping inside the white wrist cuffs. The Nurse, HCA or ODP will secure the neck and inner tie.

Your assistant will then drop two pair of gloves into the sterile area. It is good practice to ask if the patient has a latex allergy before donning your gloves (although this should be covered by the WHO checklist).

The closed method of donning gloves is preferred. Always have your fingers covered.
1. Use your right hand to remove the left glove.
2. Hold your left hand palm up with your fingers straight.
3. Lay the glove on your left wrist.
4. Grip the bottom cuff with your left thumb.
5. Place your right thumb inside the top cuff edge.
6. Stretch the glove over your left fingertips.
7. Pull down the glove with your finger straight.

Repeat the above procedure on the other side then pull down the glove and sleeve together to adjust the gown. Never expose the white wrist band of the gown, as this is permeable. It is important to double glove for your safety. It also reduces infection rates and allows you to change gloves during the procedure e.g. arthroplasty surgery or vascular procedures. Don't forget to do the final tie of the gown.

During the procedure hands should be at or above waist level and below shoulder level and visible at all times to avoid inadvertent contamination.

Gloves, masks and gowns must be disposed off in the clinical waste bins for incineration. When removing gowns, always ensure gloves remain inside and gown rolled from top to bottom to prevent contamination of theatre scrubs. Goggles are removed and put in sluice for cleansing.

Sample mark scheme

Offers to change into surgical scrubs and shoes	0	1	2
Dons hat and mask	0	1	2
Offers to remove jewellery and watch	0	1	
Checks patient has no latex allergy	0	1	
Opens gown and gloves	0	1	2
Uses pick and brush to clean fingers	0	1	2
Performs stages 2-7 appropriately	0	1	2
Repeats stages	0	1	
Dries hands and discards towel	0	1	
Dons gown maintaining sterility	0	1	
Dons gloves with closed technique	0	1	2
Second pair of gloves used	0	1	
Does final tie	0	1	
Removes gown, gloves, mask & goggles (if applicable) appropriately	0	1	

FOLLOW ON QUESTIONS

Q1. Why should one scrub before performing an operation?

A1.
(i) To remove debris and transient microorganisms from the nails, hands and forearms.
(ii) To reduce/minimise the resident microbial count to a minimum.
(iii) To eliminate controllable sources of contamination.

Q2. Why should one wear a mask, goggles, hat and clogs?

A2.
Mask & goggles reduce the risk & protects one from bodily fluids, blood & bony fragments. Research has shown a mask can reduce the risk of mycobacterial tuberculosis. Hats & hoods minimise the chance of hair or dead skin falling into a wound.

Q3. What is on the WHO checklist?

A3. "The World Health Organisation checklist allows health care professionals to minimise the most common and avoidable risks endangering the lives and well-being of surgical patients." It comprises of:
- "Sign in" before the induction of anaesthesia.
- "Time out" before the incision of the skin.
- "Sign out" before the patient leaves the operating room.

Q4. What types of surgical scrubs do you know?

A4.
- Aqueous scrubs containing chlorhexidine gluconate or povidone iodine.
- Alcohol rubs containing alcohol ethanol, isopropanol or n-propanol.
- Alcohol rubs containing chlorhexidine gluconate and iodophors.

Q5. What are the risk factors for developing a surgical site infection (SSI)?

A5.
- Age >65.
- ASA grade ≥ 3.
- Malnutrition.
- Radiotherapy or Steroids.
- Obesity.
- Smoking.
- Peripheral Vascular disease.
- Wound classification (see suturing a wound).

Further Reading

- *Association for Perioperative Practitioners Guidelines.*
- *AfPP 2007 Standards and Recommendations for Safe Perioperative Practice 2nd edition.*
- *NICE Guidelines on Surgical Site Infections (2008).*
- *World Health Organisation Surgical Safety Guidelines.*

Chapter	15	**Suturing Skills: Closure of a Wound**

Scenario

This 27-year-old man has presented to the A&E after injuring his arm on some broken glass. He has a 5x7 cm sized laceration with necrotic wound edges on the lateral aspect of his right forearm. As the surgical core trainee, you have been requested by the A&E consultant to suture the wound.

Important points not to miss

In this station, it is important not to assume anything. Even if the scenario states the patient is consented, draped and anaesthetised, you must demonstrate that you would check/repeat this. Vital marks can easily be missed even if you demonstrate a perfect wound closure technique. The maximum doses of local anaesthetic and ensuring safe follow-up planning may be assessed in this station.

Talk through

Suturing is a common task in the examination. However, this scenario not just assesses your ability to suture a wound but rather evaluates your ability to communicate with the patient, make a brief assessment and rationalise any relevant investigations. It will also test your knowledge of local anaesthetic agents, administer the anaesthetic, suture the wound and answer any follow on questions in the allotted time. It is therefore essential to have in your mind the step-by-step process for managing these situations, so you can run smoothly through the station and pick up all the available marks. In this scenario, the examiner is likely to play the patient and may have a foam pad strapped to their arm with a wound on it. Due to time restraints, it is most likely that the patient's arm will already be prepared and draped for you, but be prepared to do this yourself if asked.

Assessment

As in all stations in the exam, read the scenario carefully to understand exactly what your task is. When entering the room, use the alcohol gel provided and introduce yourself to the patient. Before you start with the task of closing the wound, you need to make a brief assessment of the patient and mention any investigations that you would like to arrange. In this scenario where the patient has suffered a glass injury to his arm, it is essential to assess the distal neurovascular function of that limb. You will not have time for a full assessment, but be sure to check distally for pulses/capillary refill and to check sensation in the distribution of the median/ulnar/radial nerves. The examiner may stop you once you have acknowledged the need to assess neurovascular function and suggest you to move on with the rest of the management. You should also ask about the patient's tetanus status, whether they have any allergy and state that you would like to arrange an X-Ray of the limb to check for foreign bodies.

Equipment
Due to time constraints, the correct equipment is usually provided for you and the patient is already prepared and draped. However, be prepared to clean and drape the wound if asked. Equipment that you may require includes:

- Sterile gloves and gown.
- Skin preparation solution (Iodine or Chlorhexidine in alcohol).
- Sterile drapes.
- 10ml syringe.
- Needles (1 x 21 & 1 x 25 gauge needle).
- Local anaesthetic (1% Lignocaine).
- Toothed forceps.
- Skin suture.
- Suture scissors.
- Adherent dressing.
- Gauze swabs.

Preparation
If the equipment is not already laid out for you and the patient is not prepared and draped, firstly open up a wound care pack, pour some antiseptic solution into the receptacle and open the relevant remaining equipment onto the sterile field. At this point state the need to wash your hands before donning a pair of sterile gloves.

Local anaesthetic
Firstly state that you would like to check the local anaesthetic and its expiry date. Then attach the 21G needle to the syringe and draw up the desired amount of anaesthetic. Discard this needle into a sharps bin and mount the 25G needle onto the filled syringe. At this point, if not already done for you, clean the wound using the antiseptic solution and use the drapes to create a surgical field. Administer the local anaesthetic appropriately around the wound, remembering to warn the patient before introducing the needle. Introduce the needle in a smooth motion, pull back on the plunger to ensure you that are not injecting into a vessel, and then slowly administer the local anaesthetic whilst withdrawing the needle. Repeat this step until the surgical field is anaesthetised adequately. Discard the needle into a sharps bin and state that you would now leave the anaesthetic to work for at least 5 minutes. Before starting to suture the wound, always check that the local anaesthetic has taken effect, either using a needle or pinching with toothed forceps.

Closure

It is most likely that the wound will be a clean, straight incision. If it is not, then state that you would like to debride the unhealthy wound edges to turn a 'traumatic wound' into a 'clean, surgical wound' before closing.

In this scenario, when suturing a traumatic wound, it is advisable to use interrupted sutures to close rather than a continuous suture. This is because if the wound became infected, then not only could the wound discharge between the interrupted sutures, but individual sutures could be removed to allow drainage, without opening up the whole wound. A suitable suture in this scenario would be a non-absorbable, monofilament suture material such as 4.0 Nylon.

Start at one end, and place a simple interrupted suture. Ensure your needle enters the skin at 90° and use the curve of the needle by fully pronating and supinating your wrist to ensure the wound edges are everted. Bring the needle out into the wound, grasp the needle again and repeat the same action for the other side of the wound. Take equal bites (roughly 0.5cm) either side of the wound, and ensure that they are of the same depth to avoid steps in the wound edges.

Place sutures roughly 1cm apart along the remainder of the wound, until it is closed adequately. Finish by applying a simple adherent dressing to the wound.

Post-operative instructions & follow up

Once you have finished the procedure, the first thing you should do is discard your sharps into a sharps bin, which will be provided in the station. At this point the patient may ask you a few questions regarding post-op instructions, but you will appear far more professional if you offer this information without being prompted. Explain that the patient will go home with some simple analgesia, and that they must seek medical attention if they are concerned about any of the following signs/symptoms:

- Increased pain.
- Redness.
- Discharge/blood through the dressing.
- Malodour.
- Systemic symptoms (fever/nausea/malaise).

Give the patient the appropriate follow-up information with regards to when and where the sutures must be removed (see Chapter 12 - 'Removing a Naevus' for timing of suture removal).

Sample mark scheme

Introduction, confirmation of patient identity	0	1	2
Professionalism	0	1	
Checks tetanus status and allergies	0	1	2
Offers X-ray to assess for foreign bodies	0	1	
Checks distal neurovascular function	0	1	2
Gathers appropriate equipment	0	1	
Applies surgical preparation	0	1	
Washes hands	0	1	
Dons gloves	0	1	
Drapes wound	0	1	
Checks local anesthetic is in date and appropriate concentration	0	1	
Checks arm is anaesthetised	0	1	
Surgical toilet with saline	0	1	
Sutures at appropriate intervals and depth	0	1	2
Gives appropriate wound care advise	0	1	2

FOLLOW ON QUESTIONS

Q1. What different types of sutures do you know?

A1. Sutures can be classified as being either natural or synthetic, braided or monofilament and absorbable or non-absorbable. It is these features that determine which sutures are used for each purpose. Examples include:

- Nylon – synthetic, monofilament, non-absorbable. Commonly used for skin closure.
- Prolene (Polypropylene) – synthetic, monofilament, non-absorbable. Used for vascular anastomosis and skin closure.
- Vicryl (Polyglactin) – synthetic, braided, absorbable (1month tensile strength, 2/12 absorbed). Used for deep closure of wounds.
- PDS (Polydioxanone) – synthetic, monofilament, absorbable (6 weeks tensile strength, 6 months absorbed). Used for tendon repairs.
- Monocryl (Poliglecaprone) – synthetic, monofilament, absorbable (2 weeks tensile strength, 3-4months absorbed). Used for subcuticular skin closure.

Q2. When is tetanus toxoid / tetanus immunoglobulin indicated?

A2. There are specific guidelines on tetanus prophylaxis for each hospital but in general wound are considered high risk if they:
- are contaminated with farmyard material such as soil or manure.
- involve the axilla or Feet.
- penetrate into the deep tissues.
- are animal or human bites.
- have large amounts of devitalised tissue.

Status	Low Risk	High Risk
Full Course with Booster < 10 years ago	Nil	Single Ig
Full Course with Booster >10 years ago	Booster Toxoid	Single Ig and Booster Toxoid
No Immunisation / Un-known	Full Course of Toxoid	Single Ig and Full Course Toxoid

Table 15.1: Tetanus status and indication for tetanus toxoid / tetanus immunoglobulin

Both toxoid and immunoglobulin are given intramuscularly and if administered at the same time must be injected at different sites. If you are concerned or unsure, mention that you would check local guidelines and discuss with the hospital microbiologist.

Q3. When would you prescribe antibiotics and for how long?

A3. The need for antibiotics depends on the nature and timing of the injury:

Type of wound	Description	Antibiotic requirement
Clean	Clean/non infected skin. GU/Resp/GI tracts not breached	None
Clean-contaminated	May breach hollow viscus but not GI tract, therefore minimal contamination. Traumatic wounds <6hrs old	Single dose
Contaminated	Breached GI tract, or traumatic wounds >6hrs old	3 doses
Dirty	Perforated viscus, heavily contaminated wounds, presence of frank pus	Prolonged antibiotics (course dependant on response)

In this scenario, the patient would need at least a single dose of antibiotic. If there was a delay in presentation, two further doses would be required post closure. For the type of antibiotic prescribed, you should follow hospital/department guidelines where available. In this clinical scenario a broad-spectrum antibiotic such as Co-amoxiclav is appropriate.

Further Reading

- *Intercollegiate Basic Surgical Skills: Course manual.*
- *NICE Guidelines on Surgical Site Infections (2008).*
- *AfPP 2007 Standards and Recommendations for Safe Perioperative Practice 2nd edition.*
- *World Health Organisation Surgical Safety Guidelines.*

Chapter 16   Knots and Tying at Depth

Scenario
You are assisting your consultant in a right hemi-colectomy and he asks you to tie-off the mesentery he's holding in a clip. Tie a braided absorbable simple reef-knot.

Important points not to miss
There is less scope for marks for preparation in this station and it will soon become apparent if you are not familiar with knot tying. So practise these techniques beforehand: in theatre, in your spare time with spare lengths of suture (or string!) or by using hand tying jigs in your clinical skills lab. In the exam, make sure your knots are firm, but avoid excess tension in order to avoid 'sawing' through the 'tissues'.

Talk through
You will be asked to demonstrate various knots using a hand tying jig and then more advanced suturing techniques on a foam pad. A patient is not usually present for this exercise.

Tie a braided absorbable simple reef-knot
The reef knot consists of two throws: the coming down and going up throw.
To start with, the coming down throw:

- Pick up the end furthest away from you (the shortest end or the white end in this example) with your left thumb and ring finger. Then lay the suture over your index and middle fingers (*Figure 16.1*).
- Using your right hand pick up the other (red) end and lay it up over the left middle and index fingers (*Figure 16.2*).
- Bend (flex) the left middle finger under the white end (*Figure 16.3*) and straighten again so that the white end is behind the middle finger under tension (*Figure 16.4*). Keep the red end under tension with your right hand.
- Now release the white end and draw it through the loop with fingers of your left hand (*Figure 16.5*).
- Lay the knot using some tension (*Figure 16.6*).

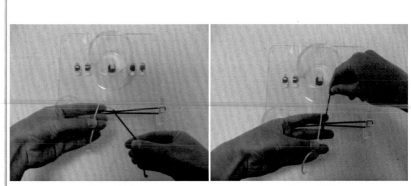

Figure 16.1   Figure 16.2

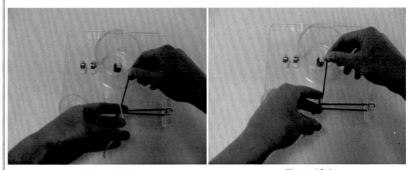

Figure 16.3   Figure 16.4

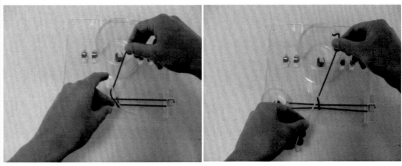

Figure 16.5   Figure 16.6

Going up throw:

- You have finished with the ends lying 180 degrees from where they started. This time pick up the white end with your left hand but direct it upwards over your little, ring and middle fingers. (*Figure 16.7*).
- With your right hand bring the red throw over the same fingers in a downwards direction (*Figure 16.8*).
- Bend (flex) your left middle finger towards you – picking up the red end (*Figure 16.9*) – and then straighten (extend) your finger back against the white end (*Figure 16.10*).
- Release the white end and draw it through the loop (*Figure 16.11*). Keep tension on the red end with the right hand.
- Lay the knot using some tension (*Figure 16.12*).

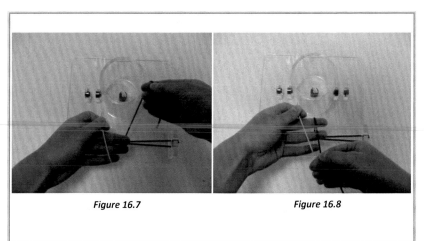

Figure 16.7   Figure 16.8

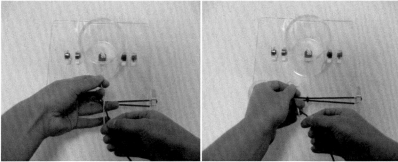

Figure 16.9   Figure 16.10

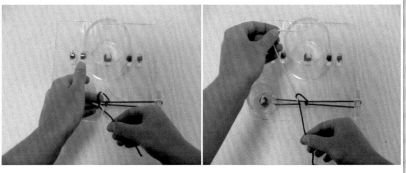

Figure 16.11   Figure 16.12

Tie a non-absorbable monofilament surgeon's knot

The examiner may ask you how to prevent a knot slipping between throws. This is your opportunity to demonstrate the surgeon's knot. This uses a double throw before laying the knot down. The key is laying the two ends over your fingers the correct way before starting.

- Grasp the end furthest away from you (the white end) between your thumb and ring finger of the left hand and lay it downwards over your fingers. Grasp the closer end (the red end) between your index finger and thumb of the right hand and lay it upwards over your fingers (*Figure 16.13*).
- Simultaneously bend (flex) both middle fingers to catch the suture, then straighten the fingers out so that the suture is on the back of each middle finger (*Figure 16.14*).
- Draw the ends of the suture through the loops you have created (*Figure 16.15*).
- Lay the knot using some tension (*Figure 16.16*).
- Tie a further single throw over to secure the knot (*Figure 16.17*).

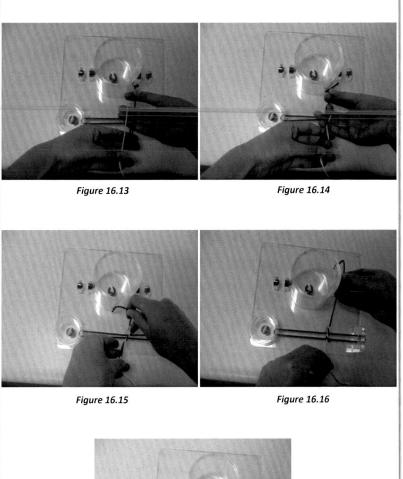

Figure 16.13

Figure 16.14

Figure 16.15

Figure 16.16

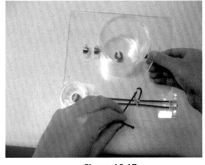

Figure 16.17

Tie an absorbable braided knot at depth

Though the throws are the same for a reef knot, your hands have to move in the vertical plane to tie at depth. This can be tricky when operating and the difficulty is replicated by using a narrow cup on the hand tying jig in the exam.

- Pass a suture around the hook (*Figure 16.18*) and tie the first throw of a reef knot (*Figure 16.19*).
- Lay the knot by pushing down with the index finger of your left hand and lifting the suture vertically with your right hand (*Figure 16.20*).
- Tie your second throw of a reef knot (*Figure 16.21* and *Figure 16.22*).
- Lay the knot using your index finger again to put the knot under tension (*Figure 16.23*).

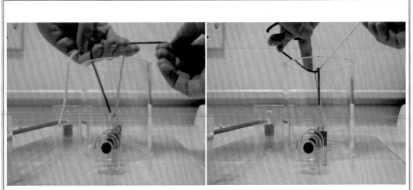

Figure 16.18

Figure 16.19

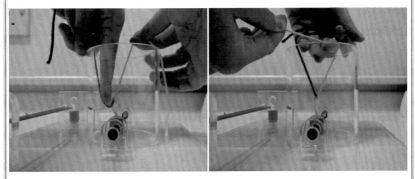

Figure 16.20

Figure 16.21

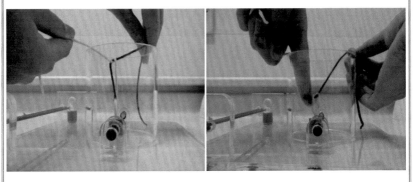

Figure 16.22

Figure 16.23

Perform a haemostatic suture for bleeding tissue using an absorbable braided suture

Surgical bleeding can be dealt with in a number of ways (pressure, diathermy, tying off of a vessel), but a Z stitch (*Figure 16.24*) is what is required by the examiner in this part of the station. This useful manoeuvre tamponades the bleeding tissue using a suture in two passes. You will need to use instruments for this part of station and demonstrate safe handling of the sharp needle.

- Angle the needle perpendicular to the tissue, to one side of the bleeding area.
- Pass the suture through the tissue and re-mount the needle.
- Aim to put the next suture on the other side of the bleeding tissue, through the tissue in the same direction as the first pass.
- Tie the two ends of the suture under some tension.

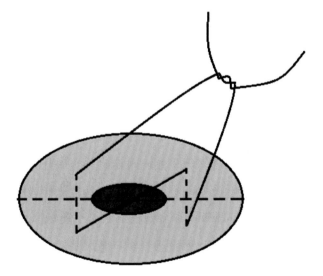

Figure 16.24

Mark Scheme

Reef knot: Familiarity	0	1	
Reef knot: Economy of movement	0	1	2
Reef knot: Secure knot	0	1	
Surgeon's knot: Familiarity	0	1	2
Surgeon's knot: Secure knot	0	1	2
Tying at depth: Initial reef knot	0	1	2
Tying at depth: Lays reef knot adequately	0	1	2
Tying at depth: Lays second reef knot (secure knot)	0	1	
Haemostatic stitch: Recognises appropriate stitch to use	0	1	2
Haemostatic stitch: Safe handling of sharps	0	1	2
Haemostatic stitch: Avoids excess tension on tissues	0	1	
Haemostatic stitch: Secure knot	0	1	2

FOLLOW ON QUESTIONS

Q1. What are the essential features of any suture?

A1. Sutures must be sterile, pliable and free of any impurities which would cause tissue to react. According to suture type, they must be of uniform size, diameter and strength.

Q2. What is meant by tensile strength and absorption?

A2. Tensile strength is a measure of the ability of the suture to resist deformation and breakage. Absorption describes the progressive loss of mass of the suture material. It does not correlate with initial tensile strength.

Q3. What different types of sutures do you know?

A3. See Chapter 15, page 83.

Q4. How are sutures classified by size?

A4. The universal system for classifying suture sizes was set up by the United States Pharmacopeia in 1937. They were originally manufactured ranging in size from #1 to #6, with #1 being the smallest. As technology improved, #0 was added to the suture diameters, and later, thinner and thinner threads were manufactured. The diameter of the suture is referred to as a number of zeroes. The greater number of zeroes, the smaller the diameter, e.g., 6-0 (0.07 mm) is smaller than 2-0 (0.30 mm). The tensile strength is directly proportional to diameter size.

Q4. What different types of needles do you know?

A4. Needles are described as having an eye (or swage), body and point. Variations in each component create differences in length, shape and needlepoint geometry. For example, differences in needlepoint distinguish tapered from cutting needles. Tapered needles are used throughout most body tissues (bowel, fascia or muscle), whereas cutting needles are used for tougher tissues such as skin, bone and tendon. Blunt-point needles can be used to close the rectus sheath in abdominal closure. Examples of variation of the needle body include:

- Straight-body needle – can be used to suture tissue that can be manipulated by hand e.g., skin closure in abdominal wounds.
- 3/8" circle curved needle – most commonly used for skin closure.
- ½" circle curved needle – for use in confined spaces e.g., deeper fascia.
- Compound curved needle i.e., different curvature at the tip compared to the body – for ophthalmic or microvascular surgery.

Further Reading

Intercollegiate Basic Surgical Skills: Course manual

Chapter 17   **Transfer Documentation**

Scenario

You are the core trainee in trauma and orthopaedic surgery at a district general hospital. A 24-year-old motor cyclist has been involved in a road traffic accident. He has sustained a closed pelvic fracture and an open tibial fracture to his right leg. He is awaiting transfer to the major trauma centre for definitive care.

1. Please read the patients notes and complete the transfer documentation.
2. Please call the receiving orthopaedic consultant to hand over the patient.

Important points not to miss

Read the notes carefully and slowly. It is essential that you have a structure to your referral whether on the phone or written. Identify yourself early and take details of the receiving team including name, rank, contact number and who else to contact if they are not available. You may not be provided with all the details that the receiving team want. Don't be tempted to make it up. This is a patient safety and probity issue and if you don't know or can't remember simply say..... "I am not 100% sure about those details, once we are off the phone I will find them out and ring you straight back." It also sounds very professional if at the end of your conversation you ask if there is anything else the receiving team would like you to do, and, if there is, make a note of it.

Talk through

General Principles

As the referring doctor, you are responsible for:

1. Initiating transfer.
2. Selecting appropriate method of transfer e.g. Helicopter, Road Ambulance.
3. Dictating the level of care en route e.g. nurse escort, technician, paramedic crew or intensive care team.

It is essential to write in a logical and structured way. Using the ATLS structure can be extremely helpful and ensures that you do not miss anything important. Offer to fax and send a copy of your documentation with the patient.

Transfer documentation structure

1. Patient Details:
    a. Name.
    b. Date of birth.
    c. Address.

2. Referrer's Details:
    a. Doctors Name.
    b. Overseeing Consultant.
    c. Hospital.
    d. Contact details e.g. Bleep Number.

3. Receiving Details:
    a. Doctors Name.
    b. Overseeing Consultant.
    c. Hospital.
    d. Contact details e.g. Bleep Number.

4. AMPLE History:
    a. Allergies.
    b. Medications.
    c. Previous Medical History.
    d. Last ate or drank.
    e. Events (put this first as it is most relevant) e.g.
        • 37-year-old male motor cyclist.
        • head on impact vs lorry at (time) on (date).
        • Combined speed 60mph.
        • Unresponsive at scene.
        • Roadside intubation .

5. ABCDE (observations):
    a. Airway - Patent, Intubated.
    b. Breathing - RR, Sats, O_2 Requirements.
    c. Circulation - HR, BP, Stable or Unstable.
    d. Disability – GCS.
    e. Exposure – Temp.

6. Probable Diagnoses:
    a. Most significant to least significant.

7. Diagnostics:
    a. Bloods.
    b. Trauma Series.
    c. CT (attach copies).

8. Treatment instituted so far:
   a. Medications – Analgesia, Anaesthetic agents, Antibiotics, Tetanus.
   b. Interventions – Chest Drains, Catheters, Access, Wound dressings.
   c. Fluids – Colloids/Crystalloids/Blood products, Volume and Timing.
9. Management during Transfer:
   a. Leave space to allow paramedics/doctor escorts to add information.

Sample mark scheme

Legible handwriting	0	1	2
Patient details included – Name, Date of Birth, Address, Hospital ID	0	1	2
Time and date of summary	0	1	
Clear documentation of receiving team/institution	0	1	
Clinical details accurate and concise			
History surrounding event/pre-hospital care	0	1	2
Past medical/surgical history	0	1	
Drug history	0	1	
Last ate/drank	0	1	
Initial assessment (structured format)	0	1	2
Diagnosis (including radiological findings/blood parameters – include copies)	0	1	
Management to date	0	1	2
Reason for transfer	0	1	
Refrained from using abbreviations	0	1	
Name and contact details of discharging doctor/consultant	0	1	2

Q1. What is a Major Trauma Centre?

A1. A single site that offers all major specialist services relevant to the care of major trauma

- General Surgery.
- Emergency medicine.
- Vascular Surgery.
- Orthopaedic Surgery.
- Plastics Surgery.
- Neurosurgery.
- Maxillofacial Surgery.
- Cardiothoracic Surgery.
- Interventional radiology.
- Critical Care.

The Royal College of Surgeons also suggests that each centre should admit a minimum of 250 critically injured patients per year.

Q2. What is the definition of major trauma?

A2. NHS Choice defines Major Trauma as multiple, serious injuries that could result in disability or death. It has previously been described as a patient with an Injury Severity Score (ISS) >15.

Further Reading

- *Advance Trauma Life Support Student handbook. American College of Surgeons Committee on Trauma. Edition 7.*

Chapter 18 — Trauma Chest Drain Insertion

Scenario

You are the surgical core trainee attending a Trauma call. This gentleman has broken ribs and a right sided pneumothorax (you will be shown an X-ray). The A&E consultant has asked you to insert a trauma chest drain.

Important points not to miss

Inserting a chest drain and answering questions regarding the management of a traumatic haemothorax or pneumothorax is a big ask for a 10 minute station so you need to ensure you know the procedure well. Have a method to assess a chest X-ray that will not miss anything (see further reading). The examiner may attempt to sway you into inserting a small-bore drain; do not go along with him/her. Knowing the key indications for insertion/referral is important and the mechanics of an underwater drain may be discussed.

Talk through

Traumatic chest drain insertion is an increasingly common exam station. You may be asked to insert a chest drain while interacting with an actor. You will be expected to obtain informed consent, undertake the procedure and answer questions about ward-based care and removal.

Indications
- Traumatic pneumothorax.
- Tension pneumothorax (post needle decompression).
- Traumatic haemothorax.
- Post-operative e.g. Thoracotomy.

Consent
- Pain.
- Scarring.
- Infection.
  - Superficial.
  - 2% risk of empyema.
- Visceral damage.
  - Cardiac.
  - Subdiaphragmatic.
- Nerve damage.
  - Intercostal neuralgia.
- Long thoracic nerve injury causing scapular winging.

- Blood vessel damage.
  - ‣ Intercostal vessel damage can convert pneumothorax to heamothorax.
- Failure of procedure.
  - ‣ Incorrect positioning.
  - ‣ Tube blockage.
  - ‣ Persistent pneumothorax.
- Recurrence post removal.
- Allergic reaction to anaesthetic or surgical preparation.

Equipment
You may be asked to select appropriate kit from a selection and place blade on scalpel using a haemostatic clamp. Immediately remove and discard the large trocar in the sterile kit!

- Sterile gloves and gown.
- Skin preparation solution (iodine or chlorhexidine in alcohol).
- Sterile drapes.
- 10ml Syringe.
- Needles (21–25 gauge).
- Gauze swabs.
- Local anaesthetic (1% or 2% lignocaine).
- Scalpel and No. 11 blade.
- Suture material (1 silk).
- Large haemostat or Spencer-Wells Clamp for blunt dissection.
- Large bore chest tube (24 to 30 French).
- Connecting tubing.
- Closed drainage system (underwater seal).
- Occlusive dressing (sleek tape).

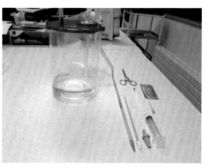

Figure 18.11: Chest Drain Equipment

Positioning
Patients should be supine with 30° of head up if possible and the bed slightly rotated towards the side of insertion. The patient's arm should be placed behind their head to expose the axillary area. It is essential that the patient undergoes regular haemodynamic observations and pulse oximetry during the procedure.

Insertion Site
Although variations have been suggested, the 'safe triangle' for insertion of a chest drain has the following borders:

- Posterior Margin - Mid-Axillary line (some literature states the anterior border of latissimus dorsi to be the posterior margin but if this is taken as a landmark, then the insertion point will be in the mid-axillary line where the long thoracic nerve lies).
- Anterior Margin - Lateral border of Pectoralis Major.
- Inferior margin - 5th intercostal space (above 6th rib).
- Apex – Below the axilla.

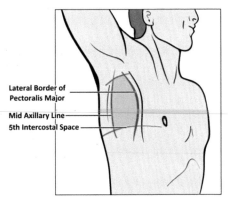

Lateral Border of Pectoralis Major

Mid Axillary Line

5th Intercostal Space

Figure 18.12: Chest Drain Insertion: The safe triangle for insertion

Ideal placement should be just anterior to the midaxillary line within this triangle to avoid damage to the long thoracic nerve of Bell. Blunt dissection should be over the superior aspect of the inferior rib in order to avoid damage to the intercostal neurovascular bundle.

Aseptic Technique
The British Thoracic Society (BTS) suggest prophylactic antibiotics for all trauma chest drain insertions. While transfer to theatre is unnecessary, sterile gloves, gown and equipment must be used. Alcoholic antiseptic solution is applied starting at the area of insertion and moving outwards. Drape the area of insertion.

Anaesthesia
Lignocaine or similar is infiltrated to the skin and periosteum of the superior margin of the inferior rib. There is no evidence that local anaesthetic with adrenaline reduces the risk of iatrogenic haemothorax. The skin is tested before any incision is made. Despite local anaesthetic the procedure is poorly tolerated by patients and concomitant anxiolytics or opiates are recommended by the BTS.

Insertion
Make a skin incision parallel and just above the rib below, slightly longer than the tube diameter (1French is 1/3mm). Use a large haemostat or clamp to blunt dissect through the parietal pleura before doing a finger sweep. A small clamp can be attached to the end of the tube through one of the holes to guide placement. Aim the tube apically for pneumathoraces and basally for haemathoraces. Watch for tube fogging to confirm appropriate placement.

Suture the drain in place with a stay suture and pass a horizontal mattress closing suture but leave this untied.

The end of the closing suture can be covered in sleek or a transparent adhesive dressing with the drain to stop it coming loose.

Drainage
A unidirectional closed drainage system such as the underwater seal drain is most commonly used. Connection tubing is used between the chest tube and underwater drain. Before the procedure is completed it is essential to ensure that the fluid within the tube is moving with respiration ("swinging" or bubbling).

Post Procedure
It is essential to obtain a chest X-ray to ensure appropriate tube placement.

Record
- Date and time of placement.
- Aseptic technique and preparation used.
- Amount and concentration of local anaesthetic.
- Tube size.
- Suture used for closure.
- Position on X-ray.
- Monitor haemodynamic status and pulse oximetry.

Removal
Removal of a chest drain can be considered when there is radiographic evidence of re-expansion and the drain has stopped bubbling. A bubbling drain should NEVER be removed.

Clamping chest drains is not recommended unless under direct supervision by a thoracic surgeon. There is no evidence that clamping a drain prior to removal reduces recurrence and it may convert a leaking drain into a tension pneumothorax.

Drains are removed during expiration or while the patient performs the Valsalva's manoeuvre. The closing suture is tied and the wound is dressed. Post removal of the drain a delayed chest X-ray should be performed.

Indications for contacting thoracic surgeons
- Pneumothorax.
  ‣ A persistent pneumothorax despite drainage may suggest a bronchial tear.

- Haemothorax.
  - More than 1,500 mL of blood immediately evacuated by tube thoracostomy.
  - Persistent bleeding 150 mL/h to 200 mL/h for 2 hours to 4 hours.
  - Persistent blood transfusion is required to maintain hemodynamic stability.

Sample mark scheme

Introduction, confirmation of patient identity	0	1	2
Consent	0	1	2
Positioned patient with arm over head	0	1	
Identifies "triangle of safety"			
5th intercostal space	0	1	
Anterior to midaxillary line	0	1	
Lateral to Pectoralis Major	0	1	
Prepared and Draped	0	1	
Local anaesthetic infiltrated	0	1	
2-3cm transverse incision over rib	0	1	
Blunt dissection through parietal pleura	0	1	
Tube advanced without trocar	0	1	
Connects to underwater seal apparatus	0	1	
Purse string suture	0	1	2
Dressing	0	1	
Post procedure instructions			
Chest X-ray	0	1	
ABG or Oximetry	0	1	
Remove drain once lung fully expanded	0	1	

FOLLOW ON QUESTIONS

Q1. What are the indications for a trauma chest drain?

A1.
- Traumatic pneumothorax.
- Tension pneumothorax (post needle decompression).
- Traumatic haemothorax.
- Post-operative e.g. thoracotomy.

Q2. What are the borders of the "safe triangle"?

A2.
- Posterior Margin - Mid-axillary line.
- Anterior Margin - Lateral Border of Pectoralis Major.
- Inferior margin - 5th Intercostal Space
- Apex – Below the axilla.

Q3. What size chest tube is appropriate for adult trauma patients?

A3. Large bore chest tube (24 to 30 French).

Q4. What are the complications of placing a trauma chest drain?

A4.
- Pain.
- Scarring.
- Infection.
- Visceral damage.
- Nerve damage.
- Blood vessel damage.
- Failure of procedure.
- Recurrence of pneumothorax or haemothorax post removal.
- Allergic reaction to anaesthetic or surgical preparation.

Q5. When should a chest drain be clamped?

A5.

Clamping chest drains is not recommended unless under the direct supervision of a thoracic surgeon. A bubbling chest drain should NEVER be clamped!

Q6. When should you contact a Thoracic Surgeon for help?

A6.

Emergency contact is suggested for haemathoraces with:

- More than 1,500 mL of blood immediately evacuated by tube thoracostomy.
- Persistent bleeding 150 mL/h to 200 mL/h for 2 hours to 4 hours.
- Persistent blood transfusion is required to maintain hemodynamic stability.

Pneumothorax

- A persistent pneumothorax despite drainage may suggest a bronchial tear.

Further Reading

- *Advance Trauma Life Support Student handbook. American College of Surgeons Committee on Trauma. Edition 7 .*

| Chapter | 19 | **Writing a Discharge Summary** |

Scenario
In your exam you may be asked to write a discharge summary or referral letter for your patient. This will be a station with minimal interaction with an examiner and although it may seem easy, time will be against you when hunting through a complex set of notes.

Important points not to miss
You must remember the key components of any medical document. Your handwriting should be legible, and information should be clear and concise. Avoid the use of abbreviations, and both patient and staff details should be clearly displayed. The ten minutes allowed for this station might go very quickly so get the important details down early. Although scoring vital marks may appear to be easy in this station, you may struggle if you are complacent and have not given this station enough thought beforehand. You may run the risk of time pressure, and consequently, forget vital information.

Talk through
You may be provided with a small set of case notes and given a pencil and paper. From the notes you can find out all patient details, the course of events during their admission and instructions for post discharge follow up. The written instructions will ask you to:
1.   Write a letter to a GP explaining how a patient's warfarin is to be managed post-operatively.
2.   Write a discharge letter to the GP for this patient who has just had a mastectomy and suffered a post-operative seroma. She is going to stay with her daughter so the letter is for her daughter's GP.

Start by reading through the patient notes briefly. There will almost certainly be some key point that will need to be included such as a surgical complication or the initiation of a new medication that may interfere with warfarin. Make sure you fill in all of the appropriate boxes. The GP details can usually be found at the front of the patient's notes or on an A&E proforma. Admission and discharge dates can be found easily and it is important to ensure appropriate follow-up is requested. This may be found on the operation note or somewhere in the post-op medical documentation.

Sample mark scheme

Legible handwriting	0	1	2
Patient details included – Name, Date of Birth, Address, Hospital ID, Telephone number	0	1	2
Time and date of summary	0	1	2
Clear documentation of receiving team/institution	0	1	2
Clinical details accurate and concise			
Diagnosis	0	1	
Procedure	0	1	2
Post-procedure events	0	1	2
Follow up required/any instructions to give	0	1	2
Medication details	0	1	2
No abbreviations	0	1	
Name and contact details of discharging doctor	0	1	2

FOLLOW ON QUESTIONS

There are no follow on questions for this station as the examiner will take your discharge summary for marking and will not interact with you.

Further Reading

- GMC Guidelines: Good Medical Practice (2012).

Index